Unveiling
the Secrets of the
Gut-Brain Connection

Unlocking Your Gut's Potential:
A Practical Guide to Healing,
Reducing Stress, Enhancing Sleep,
and Embracing a Happier, Healthier
You!

Marusya Wellness Publishing

Contents

Introduction

Tell me what you eat and I will tell you who you are.
–Jean Anthelme Brillat-Savarin.

If you were asked, "Which organ is most closely linked to your feelings?" you would probably give one of two answers: Your brain or your heart. Nobody would think to say "my gut." After all, your gut isn't really related to your feelings, right? Well, that's not entirely true. It plays a far bigger role in how you feel on a day-to-day basis—and in your overall health and well-being—than you'd think. For instance, did you know that "serotonin" (otherwise known as the happiness hormone) is actually stored in your gut, as opposed to your brain? It's true! In fact, your gut is responsible for providing 95% of the total serotonin your body produces (Appleton, 2018).

That's a whole lot of happiness when you think about it! But your happiness isn't the only thing your gut plays an unexpected role in. Your gut activity also influences the quality and duration of your sleep, sensitivity to pain, general appetite, and mood. In short, it's vital for your ability to lead a healthy and happy life. It's interesting, then, that there are so many of us around that are neither very happy nor all that healthy. Various health issues, be they physical or mental, have been on the rise for a few decades now and show little to no signs of stopping or slowing down. One example is obesity, which is one of the leading health problems around the world and is certainly a major issue in the US. Since 1975, worldwide obesity has all but tripled, and surveys indicate that there were 1.9 billion obese adults across the globe in 2016. Meanwhile, 39 million children were diagnosed with obesity in 2020 (*Obesity and Overweight*, 2021).

Obesity is clearly a major problem around the world, but it's not the only one. Cases of diabetes and depression have been steadily climbing over the years as well, as a quick look at the most recent health statistics would show you. Between 1988 and 2004, the number of diabetic people across the globe took a staggering jump from 108 million to 422 million. Diabetes was the main cause of death for 2 million different individuals in 2019 alone (*Diabetes*, 2023). As for depression, it's estimated that about 280 million people around the world are currently struggling with this mental health disorder, and more than 700,000 people commit suicide because of it every year.

Given the role that the gut plays in mood management and digestion, it can easily be said that your gut health has a lot to do with your experiencing such health problems. Furthermore, it can be said that the way people have been managing (or mismanaging) their gut health is at least partly responsible for the unexplained surge in digestive issues, mental health issues, obesity, diabetes, and even neurodivergent issues we have been seeing since the 1700s.

If we want to understand such issues and find a way to resolve them, then we have to understand that neither the gut nor the brain can be considered separately. Instead, they must be considered as parts of a whole that influence and impact each others' responses and reactions. In this sense, our bodies can be compared to an ecosystem. In an ecosystem, different forces of nature directly impact one another. If one is off balance, all other forces become off balance as well, which messes with the well-being of the ecosystem. The same thing happens with our bodies. That being the case, is it really all that surprising to find out that your gut health can influence your other organs, such as your brain, and play a determining role in your general health?

Our body is a complex system, with different components interacting with each other on a daily basis. When it comes to our health, it's important to keep this in mind. This fact is something that scientists and researchers had a hard time grasping for a while. That's why many were greatly surprised to discover the inextricable link between our guts and brains. However, once this link was discovered, it was undeniable. What's more, it was so strong that scientists ended up giving a brand new moniker to the human gut: The second brain.

Unfortunately, while the gut is vital in our ability to maintain our physical and mental health, this link is still something that a great many of us are unaware of. This means that there are a lot of people trying to figure their way out of various health problems without realizing that a significant number of their issues could be solved by improving their gut health. They don't realize, for instance, that various mental health issues can be solved (or at least better managed) by changing their diet or taking medication that can balance out their gut microbiome.

However, if you've picked up The Gut-Brain Connection, you're not one of these people. Instead, you're among the select few that realize they must carefully consider their gut health to improve their overall health and well-being. This is exactly what you'll be learning how to do throughout this book. In doing so, you'll finally come to grasp the nexus between the gut, brain, and general health. You'll then be able to achieve an optimal level of health by simply making a few minor adjustments to your diet and lifestyle.

Chapter 1:
The Brain-Gut Microbiome (BGM) Axis

First things first—what exactly is a microbiome? It can be described as the general collection of microorganisms populating a particular area of your body, in this case, your gut (Microbiome, 2019). These microorganisms are things like bacteria, which aren't all bad. In fact, some bacteria are very good for you and your digestive system, and you want more of these in your gut. This is because the microorganisms making up your gut biome play a crucial role in your gut health and, thus, your general health and well-being, as you'll soon see. Not only that, but they also influence your "gut feeling," which, contrary to what you might think, is a very real thing.

A History of the BGM Axis

Have you ever heard of or said the phrase, "I have a gut feeling about this"? If so, then the gut feeling(also known as intuition) is something you're acquainted with. You might think that associating intuitive feelings with your gut is a bit odd, but in reality, it makes a great deal of sense. This is because your gut microbiome has the power and ability to alter your brain chemistry (Carpenter, 2012). In doing so, it can cause you to become very anxious, quite brave, and anything in between.

Those are actual feelings that come from your brain, though. So what are gut feelings precisely, and what do they really feel like? A lot of different kinds of sensations count as "gut feelings." For example, a sudden outbreak of goosebumps or butterflies in your stomach is a gut feeling. So is a sinking sensation in your stomach, sweaty hands, and an unexpected flash of clarity and calm (Raypole, 2021). These are all sensations that you feel intuitively, and they all come from your gut.

So, how and why do gut feelings emerge? Why does the gut have the power to influence your mood and feelings, to begin with? To understand this, you first have to grasp the nature of the connection between the gut and the brain and how it works. The gut-brain connection, otherwise known as the gut-brain axis (BGM), has only recently gained attention from neurologists, nutritionists, and microbiologists. However, this connection has existed for a long time. Until recently, scientists viewed different organ systems, such as the digestive and nervous systems, as separate entities that did not affect each other. This is why the idea of the BGM has only recently gained attention as a topic of discussion.

Scientists got their first inkling that there might be a connection between the gut and the brain in the 18th century. This was thanks to a scientist called Paul Joseph Barthez, who observed that organs such as the heart and the stomach preserve their level of activity far longer than other organs do when they're cut off from regular blood flow (Lewandowska-Pietruszka et al., 2022). This observation prompted the question of why and made some scientists look closer at the gut. One such scientist was Robert Whytt, who discovered that the gut is home to several nerve endings. It was upon this discovery that Whytt coined the term "nervous sympathy," thereby introducing the concept that all organs within the body(including the brain and gut) are connected and part of a single, comprehensive communications network (Nguyen & Palm, 2022).

With the introduction of "nervous sympathy," scientists adopted a far more holistic approach to human health. Because of this, they learned that the gastrointestinal tract (GI tract) has over 100 million nerve endings, not just a few. These nerve endings primarily make it possible for us to digest food without thinking about it, much like how our hearts beat without conscious thought. Remember those gut feelings like butterflies in your stomach? Well, it turns out that these nerve endings are why you have them too. This is because they make the GI tract sensitive to all sorts of emotions, be it elation, stress, anger, fear, or something else entirely. They are to blame for the stomachaches and cramps you get when you're stressed, as these result from the GI nerve endings responding to what you're feeling.

The thing about GI tract nerve endings is that they, by nature of their location, come into direct contact with the food and beverages you consume. This means that they can be affected by these things in some major ways. Drinking too much tea or alcohol, for example, can cause digestion issues and emotional struggles, thanks to how they affect those nerves. When you consider how the food you consume impacts your gut microbiota, those effects are only heightened.

Like nervous sympathy, the gut microbiota was first thrust into the spotlight in the 19th century. In 1842, a man called John Goodsir discovered a bacteria called Sarcina ventriculi in a patient's stomach. This kickstarted an intense debate because some scientists believed that this was a harmful bacteria that should be eliminated, while others opposed this idea. Further research led to the discovery of even more bacteria in the gut (Lewandowska-Pietruszka et al., 2022). One scientist, Theodor Escheric, later discovered that a healthy child's gut contains a kind of bacteria that's typically seen in the guts of adults who have diarrhea. This showed that the gut microbiome was much more complicated than people thought and that different microorganisms are required for good gut health.

The revelations about the gut microbiome made a lot of scientists question how it affected the nerve endings in the GI tract and, thus, emotions. In the 20th century, this became a heavy topic of discussion. For instance, one scientist, William Fenwick, stated that science couldn't answer the question of how the stomach relates to strong emotions. At the same time, various psychoanalysts drew attention to how people's emotional states affected their gastrointestinal symptoms, sometimes making them far worse. Thus, a link was drawn between stress and gastrointestinal issues and the idea that gastrointestinal ulcers occurred in people with high stress and anxiety levels.

In 1904, scientist Elie Metchnikoff stepped onto the scene with a hypothesis. According to his observations, certain microorganisms could prevent milk from souring. Based on this, he theorized that certain bacteria could also stop "intestinal putrefaction," thereby slowing down or even stopping aging. The idea caught on and later gave rise to detailed research on probiotics. Simultaneously, a man called Arthur Samuel Kendall came to the forefront. He directed people's attention to the connection between diet and microbiota composition, showing how the two influence one another. He identified a great number of microorganisms making up the gut microbiota. Still, he maintained that he couldn't possibly identify them all. He wasn't wrong. In the 1970s, scientists were able to identify 400 to 500 different microorganisms. Later, it was found that some 1000 species of microorganisms live in our guts, and identifying them all would be a massive undertaking.

Thanks to all this research, terms such as microbiota and psychobiotic rapidly caught on in the 20th century. Scientists' interest in how the gut was connected to the brain only increased as the years went by, and the more people looked, the more fascinating their findings became. For example, in 2004, scientists examined the stress responses of two different mice: One with a specific kind of bacteria in its gut and another without it. They quickly saw that the mouse without that bacteria in its system was far more sensitive to stress than the one with it (Sudo et al., 2004). Clearly, there was such a thing as the brain-gut axis. It heavily influenced both human emotions and health and well-being.

The Brain-Gut Axis

So, what exactly is the brain-gut axis, and how does it work? In layman's terms, the brain-gut axis is a two-way system between the gut and the brain that the two use to communicate and influence one another (Rege, 2019). That the axis is a two-way street means that the gut has the ability to talk to the brain, just as the brain has the ability to talk to the gut. This means that by communicating with the brain, your gut can influence your mood, behavior, brain development, immune system strength, and overall health. Likewise, the brain can regulate your digestive system and control your appetite.

The part of your nervous system that's responsible for this is called the enteric nervous system (ENS) (Rao & Gershon, 2016). If you want to get a little more specific, the ENS is a part of your autonomic nervous system, which is in charge of controlling involuntary physiological actions such as keeping your heart beating, your lungs breathing, and your gastrointestinal system working (Waxenbaum et al., 2020). Now, with that in mind, there are three components that make up your gut-brain axis: Your brain, your gut, and the microbiota coating it. Of these, your brain is the operations center of the axis. It makes all the major decisions and coordinates and controls all activities. For instance, a part of the brain called the hypothalamus actively controls your thirst and hunger, among other things, thus telling you when to drink and eat (Johnson, 2018).

Remember those 100 million nerve cells in your guts? Well, those nerve cells make your ENS (Rao & Gershon, 2016). They receive orders from your brain on how to manage things like digestion and talk back to your brain as needed. Finally, there's your microbiota. Your microbiota is made up of 100 trillion microbial cells. That means there are many different microorganisms in your gut, including bacteria, fungi, archaea, and even viruses. It's worth mentioning that a healthy gut needs these things, as not all microbial cells are bad for you. In fact, several of them are very good for you, as you'll see in the coming chapters. Aside from being very good for you, they're also quite fascinating, given the complex ways in which they can impact your health and mood. Even the most minor change to your gut microbiota can have monumental effects on these things.

The Bottom-Up and Top-Down Communication

So, how exactly is the gut connected to the brain? There's a specific nerve that's responsible for this connection, and it's known as the vagus nerve. Linking the gut directly to the brain connects both bottom-up and top-down nerves (Breit et al., 2018). Bottom-up nerves are nerves that send information from the gut to the brain. As such, they're input nerves. Top-down nerves are the very opposite of bottom-up ones. They send info from the brain down to the guts or wherever else. As such, they're output nerves.

On the whole, there are three pathways that these nerves follow to get gut information to the brain or from the brain to the gut. These are neuroendocrine pathways, neuroimmune pathways, and direct neural signaling. Let's unpack those terms for a minute. Neuroendocrine pathways are the paths your nerves use to transmit information like hormonal changes, safety-related issues, and stomach-related matters to your brain (Saranya, 2020). As part of this system, the neuroendocrine cells that line your gut create several chemicals and hormones. These then make their way into your circulation system and use that to snake their way up to your brain. Once there, they trigger a whole cascade of biochemical reactions that affect you in numerous ways.

Neuroimmune pathways are the paths used to communicate information about your immune system, as you might have guessed from its name. The way they work is relatively simple. The process starts with your gut microbiota conversing with your central nervous system, being the Chatty Cathies that they are. The information that they send to your brain is related to the strength of your immune system, how your immune cells are moving through your body, whether there's any inflammation in your gut, and if so, what the response to it is like. Having received this information, the brain can send orders down to make necessary adjustments. This pathway further plays a part in developing the immune cells found in your brain.

Last but not least, there's direct neural signaling. This is the system used to send information about things like what the food components you're digesting are, what inflammatory molecules are in your system, and what metabolites are being produced. Such information is relayed to your CNS, as before, and the brain uses what it's told to decide what it wants to do. This is why the information relayed through direct neural signaling can alter how independently your GI tract can move, how much mucus your body needs to secrete, and how much gastric acid your stomach needs to produce to digest your food.

Think of all three of these pathways as highways. Of course, you'll need a vehicle of some sort to navigate highways, and that's where the fatty acids and metabolites(which your gut microbiome directly produces) come in. These are the vehicles your nerves use to transmit whatever they need to and from your gut and your brain. This information is then used to make adjustments and respond to any adjustments that your brain requires. If you want your physical and mental health to be top-notch, then you want these pathways to communicate good information. For this to occur, it is important to maintain a healthy gut by having a well-balanced and healthy microbiota. What exactly does that mean? Let's find out!

Chapter 2:
Exploring the World of Gut
Microbes

The human body is fascinating and filled with all sorts of mind-boggling mysteries. Take your gut microbiome, for instance. Many of you may not know that this complex ecosystem of microorganisms weighs approximately 4.4 lbs (2 kilos) (Ferranti et al., 2014). This weight gives you an idea as to how many microorganisms are in your gut, given that they're too small to see unless you're looking at them under a microscope. Of course, your gut isn't the only part of your body that's host to a multitude of microorganisms. In fact, every part of your body, be it external, like your skin, or internal, like your nasal cavity, throat, or even private parts, is coated in them. They all have their own unique microbiome environments. However, your most complicated microbiome is the one in your gut in terms of both size and diversity.

Since the microbiomes in the various parts of your body have different environments, they can also have different compositions. Not only that, but the gut microbiome of one individual can vastly differ from that of another. Even different sections of your GI tract can be home to different kinds of microorganisms or have varying quantities of them. With all that being the case, it shouldn't be surprising to find out that the gut microbiome has a whole other name it goes by these days—the second human genome.

Second Human Genome

In biology, "genome" is the official term used to describe DNA, which is the full genetic information that defines who you are and what makes you "you" (Green, 2019). So, how can your gut microbiome be considered your second human genome? This has a lot to do with how genetically diverse your gut microbiome is (Grice & Segre, 2012). Every one of the microorganisms that make this ecosystem up is alive. This means that as small as they are, they have their own genetic materials, which allow them to work in very specific methods and thus impact your body in various ways. This is why your gut microbiome affects things like your immune system, metabolism, and even your body's ability to manage how certain drugs are broken down in your system.

Given the size and diversity of the gut microbiome, some scientists consider it to be a whole other organ in addition to being the second genome. After all, it has its own unique pathology and physiology and is something that can be genetically inherited. Given the number of microorganisms that knit it together, it shouldn't be surprising to hear that a lot of research still needs to be done about the gut microbiome, especially when you factor in how those organisms influence and interact with one another. Just as your various organs, like the gut and the brain, continually interact with one another, the microorganisms in your gut microbiota also constantly interact with one another. A change in the quantity of one microorganism can therefore have a ripple effect and cause major consequences—be they good or bad—as you'll see in coming chapters.

Members of the Gut Microbiota

While listing all the different organisms that knit your microbiota together is next to impossible, dividing them into certain distinct categories is possible. Overall, your gut bacteriome falls into one of three categories. These are

- prokaryotes

- eukaryotes

- viruses

You probably haven't heard of these before, except for viruses, and the idea that there could be viruses in your gut that are good for you might be strange. So, what exactly are these microorganism types, and how are they good for you? First, there are the prokaryotes. A prokaryote is a single-celled organism that doesn't have a cell membrane or any kind of specialized organelle. Typically, a bacteria would be considered a prokaryote (Marchesi, 2010). There are a lot of prokaryotes throughout the human body, not just the gut. In fact, there are so many of them that they outnumber the cells in your body ten-to-one, though there's some debate as to whether that figure could be closer to one-to-one (Kodio et al., 2020). Like viruses, you're probably used to thinking of bacteria as the bad guys. However, your gut needs certain types of bacteria to maintain its stability and health.

Then there are the eukaryotes. A eukaryote is an organism that can consist of a single cell or multiple cells. It has its own nucleus too, which contains the genetic information—DNA—specific to that organism. Archeas, fungi, and eubacterium are examples of eukaryotes (Kodio et al., 2020). Though many people have grown used to considering eukaryotes as "parasites" that need to be gotten rid of, they're essential to your gut health. For example, certain kinds of eukaryotes, known as helminths, actively help regulate your immune system (Lukeš et al., 2015). Some other kinds of eukaryotes help your gut maintain its mucus membrane, which it needs to do if you want to be able to digest food properly.

Finally, there are viruses, which aren't bad to have in your gut, contrary to what you might think. Known as gut viromes, some of these microorganisms end up in your gut through the food you consume. Others have just naturally been a part of it for a long time (Lecuit & Eloit, 2017). Your gut virome's presence is regulated by the eukaryotes in your system, and this is just one example of the different organisms of your gut interacting with one another. There are many other ways in which they communicate and play with one another, thereby affecting your body and health in a multitude of ways. How exactly did all these organisms come together to form your microbiome, though, and do they change and evolve in any way as you age?

The Development of Gut Microbiome

Everyone's gut microbiome is a little (or a lot) different from those of others. Yours is too. This is because several factors influence the development of your gut microbiome. These factors are your genes, the environment you live in, the food you eat, and any medication you may be taking (Tanaka & Nakayama, 2017). Of these, the food you eat, meaning your diet, plays a particularly important role. When you eat something, the dietary fiber inside what you've eaten gets broken down by the enzymes created by the microbiota in your colon. These microbiota then ferment that which they've broken down. This process creates a chain of short-chain fatty acids, which lowers the acidity (pH) levels of your colon. This, in turn, determines which microbiota can survive in the established acidity of the environment.

As a general rule, you want the pH levels of your colon to be low. This is because low pH levels restrict the growth and development of harmful bacteria in your gut. They also have the added benefit of stimulating your immune cells and ensuring your blood sugar and cholesterol levels remain within normal and healthy ranges. Maintaining a healthy gut microbiome depends on the food you consume. It is essential to include foods that contain resistant starches to lower colon pH levels, as well as prebiotic fibers like garlic, leeks, and other similar greens to support gut health (The Microbiome, 2017).

Though the food you eat is very important, your gut microbiome doesn't start developing the day you start eating solid foods. Instead, it begins doing so when you're a fetus in utero. Studies suggest that this process begins when you're a very young fetus and your forming body is engulfed by the amniotic fluid filling the womb you're in. This amniotic fluid, which is there to protect you, contains some bacterial strains within it. Once you absorb those strains into yourself, they make their way to your gut, where they begin propagating and forming your microbiome bit by bit (Wernroth et al., 2022).

Another thing that affects the makeup of your microbiome is your birth. The way you're delivered, such as whether your mother undergoes a natural birth or has a c-section, ultimately affects your microbiome. So does how much time you spend in the hospital following your delivery. Whether you're breastfed or given formula impacts this too, which makes sense when you think about it. Sanitation and antibiotic treatments play a part in your gut microbiota as well. This is because antibiotics can very easily eradicate certain bacterial microbiota chains, even if they're good for you. Simultaneously, they can cause others to grow overly large, which can throw your microbiota off balance (Fessl, 2022). Of course, over time, your microbiota will grow resistant to antibiotics, but that's only after it has been altered to some degree. That's why you should always take care when you're taking antibiotics. That's not to say you shouldn't take them if you really need them and have been given a prescription for them. However, it means that they shouldn't be your first resort if you want to care for your gut health.

Though the development of your gut microbiome kicks off before you're even born, your microbiome sees significant growth when you're two to three years old and becomes what it'll be like in your adulthood when you get to be five years old, assuming you don't dramatically change your diet later on, of course.

The microbiome you eventually end up with is made up of prokaryotes, eukaryotes, and viromes, as you've seen, and all of these form a sort of symbiotic relationship with you. That means that, just as they're good for you in a number of ways, you're good for them in that you provide them with the optimal living environment and the resources they need to survive. True, the microbiota do have to compete with one another for these resources, but that's to be expected of any overpopulated region, isn't it? Still, some of the microbiota aren't good for you, as you've seen, which is why it's so important you maintain the kind of healthy diet that can do away with them and feed the microbiota that are good for you.

The Good Guys vs. the Bad Guys

So, who are the good and bad guys of your gut microbiome, and how exactly do they compete for the available resources? As you know, the kind of food you eat changes the acidity of your gut. This then determines which of your microbiota can survive in the environment that has been created. The first food you ever consume will either be breast milk or formula. While sometimes babies cannot have breast milk for specific health reasons—for instance, if the mother is very sick and therefore on some strong medication—as a rule, you should opt for breast milk over formula if you can. This is because studies show that breast milk contains certain antibodies that increase your immunity to diseases, including gut infections. In addition to that, these antibodies, known as IgG, facilitate the growth of good bacteria in your gut. In doing so, they strengthen your immune system (Sanidad et al., 2022).

The thing about newborns is that their immune system isn't fully developed yet. As such, it can't prevent the bad bacteria in the gut from developing and gaining strength over the good bacteria. The antibodies in breast milk can. Therefore, babies must be given breast milk until their immune system becomes strong enough to keep the bad guys at bay and support the good guys in their gut. By doing so, they will be able to maintain a reasonable balance in their gut microbiome. Also, the good bacteria in their gut will have become healthy and strong enough to help with this. That means that the gut microbiota in your gut doesn't just offer you various health benefits. They also actively resist and fight off the bad bacteria in your gut, and they work diligently with your natural antibodies to do so.

All that being said, your gut microbiota is very susceptible to change. Change your diet in the right way, and you can support the good guys in your gut. Change it in the wrong way, and you'll be damaging your gut health quite a bit. The thing is that the food that you eat doesn't just impact your gut pH. It influences the properties of your gut walls, the composition of the mucus in your gut, and its ability to produce immunoglobulin A. The property of your gut walls is important because these walls are what your gut microbiota sticks to.

The mucus composition in your gut is also important because it has a two-way relationship with the microbiota. On one end, your gut mucus provides the microbiota with the ideal environment to survive and thrive in. On the other end, the microbiota ensures the health of the mucus layer in your gut. It helps keep it functional, and some of the bacteria in it can both improve upon it and keep it in tip-top shape. This is important because that mucus layer is good for many different things. For starters, it serves as your gut's first layer of protection. At the same time, it serves as a kind of lubricant, ensuring that the food you eat passes through your intestines without any issues. Its symbiotic relationship with your microbiota also helps fend off diseases (Paone & Cani, 2020).

Then there's immunoglobulin A (IgA). IgA is a type of antibody that's produced in mucus surfaces. Seeing as your intestines are coated in a mucus layer, it can be found there in abundance. In fact, nearly two grams of IgA are created in your gut every single day. The thing about this antibody is that it binds itself to the bacteria in the gut. In doing so, it helps shape the gut microbiome and influences how your microbiota behave. Meanwhile, it protects the gut and the gut microbiota against any toxins or pathogens you may have ingested (Yang & Palm, 2020).

What Shapes the Gut Microbiome?

So then, what exactly shapes your gut microbiome? Clearly, the kind of diet you had as an infant—breast milk vs. formula—plays a part in this, but things don't just end there. There eventually comes a time when you start eating solid foods, after all, and the food you eat plays a determinant role in shaping your microbiome too. Overall, eating greens (meaning fruits and vegetables) tends to help your gut microbiome maintain its health. The nutrients in these foods support the good bacteria and help maintain the pH balance you want. A veggie-heavy, even vegetarian diet typically results in a diverse microbiome that can metabolize carbs faster.

Sadly, most people don't maintain vegetarian or even veggie-heavy diets. The usual Western diet is a far cry from such things, as they're characterized by fast foods, greasy foods, sugar, and carbs. The problem with this kind of Western diet is that it can cause healthy bacteria (such as firmicutes, for example) to be killed off. This is problematic since firmicutes produce something called butyrate, which supports the gut lining, is an antioxidant, and helps prevent certain types of cancer, among other things (Edermaniger, 2021).

We all have those moments of weakness where we think, "It's just a cheat meal" or "It's just one day; what's the harm?" before we dig into food that we know is bad for us. The thing is, such a decision brings with it plenty of harm because even short-term changes to your diet can significantly change your microbiota makeup. This is something you need to bear in mind when you're contemplating what to eat and feel temptation calling. Overall, you should try to eat a healthy, green diet as much as you can. Contrary to what you might think, you shouldn't exclude gluten from your diet unless you have a gluten allergy or celiac disease. It must be said that a lot of research still needs to be done on the link between gluten and the gut microbiome. However, early studies indicate that removing gluten from your diet can significantly affect your gut microbiome. For instance, one study has found that the healthy and unhealthy bacteria ratios become quite unbalanced in the gut microbiome once gluten has been removed from the equation (Polo et al., 2020).

While reducing your gluten intake can have some benefits, like increasing the ratio of healthy fibers in your gut, removing them entirely seems to be a bad idea. This makes sense when you think about it. The general rule anyone who wishes to live a healthy life should abide by is that one should neither overindulge nor under indulge in things. Doing either is a prime way to throw things off balance, and you want your gut microbiome to be well-balanced if you want it to be able to serve its protective and metabolic roles properly. As a general rule, you want to ensure your gut microbiome is well-balanced. Only then can you ensure that your gut microbiota can fulfill the various metabolic and protective roles it is tasked with, as you'll soon see.

Chapter 3:

Metabolic and Protective
Roles of Gut Microbiota

Your gut microbiota offers you many benefits and serves a lot of different purposes. One of these is that it plays a part in your ability to metabolize the food and even drugs you consume. They primarily metabolize carbs and, in the process, produce substances like butyrate, which you recently learned is very good. They also play a role in lipid and protein metabolism and synthesize vitamins B and K. On top of that, they break down polyphenols and create substances that are good for you, like flavonoids, which are then absorbed by your gut (Jandhyala, 2015). These are just a few examples of the metabolic functions of your gut microbiome. It also has protective functions. Your gut microbiota plays a significant role in your mucosal immune system, which grants you antimicrobial protection and supports the production of various immune cells. To better understand all these different functions and benefits, let's take a closer look at them, starting with lipid metabolism.

Lipid Metabolism

Lipid metabolism describes how the lipids like fatty acids in meals are broken down and then stored as energy for later. The amount and kinds of lipids you consume affect your microbiota, just as your microbiota affects how those lipids are metabolized (Schoeler & Caesar, 2019). Hence, there's yet another symbiotic relationship between the two. Gut microbiota can synthesize, transform, and break down dietary lipids. In doing so, they produce certain metabolites, which are necessary for metabolism to occur.

Meanwhile, lipids that have been transformed and synthesized affect both immune pathways and metabolic ones. This means that, by maintaining a healthy diet, one can potentially avoid the development of conditions such as autoimmune diseases, chronic inflammation, and metabolic syndromes such as obesity and cardiovascular diseases (Brown et al., 2023).

One very interesting fact about gut microbiota is that it can regulate your hepatic lipid metabolism, meaning your liver's lipid metabolism capability. While how the gut microbiota achieves this isn't exactly clear yet, it is known that individuals who don't have diverse gut microbiota have slower and less efficient hepatic lipid metabolisms. It's also known that the short fatty acids that the gut microbiome produces (along with other things like bile acids, lipopolysaccharides, and microbial metabolites derived from amino-acid) help regulate lipid metabolism. It's obvious then that both the gut microbiota and the metabolites they make have a role to play in hepatic lipid metabolism (Han et al., 2022).

On top of that, the gut microbiome has some responsibility in cholesterol metabolism. Clear evidence of this is the link between it and hypercholesterolemia, which is a lipid disorder (Vourakis et al., 2021). Hypercholesterolemia is a disorder that, when left unchecked, can very easily lead to cardiovascular diseases. Studies indicate that your gut microbiome can help your cholesterol metabolism by producing useful metabolites like bile acids. These can then regulate said metabolism, thereby preventing hypercholesterolemia from ever becoming a thing and stopping cardiovascular disease before it can take root too. Even with all that being said, scientists have only just begun exploring the connection between the gut microbiome and cholesterol metabolism, so there's still much to discover. Given the sheer size of the gut microbiome, how could there not be? It's not for nothing that the gut microbiome is still being studied in a multitude of ways.

Insulin Sensitivity

Another thing your gut microbiota impacts is your insulin sensitivity. Insulin sensitivity is your cells' overall responsiveness to insulin. Generally speaking, you want to be highly sensitive to insulin because the more you are, the more you'll be able to avoid and prevent insulin-related diseases. People who are insulin-sensitive don't have insulin resistance or diabetes, for example. This is because being sensitive makes your cells better able to use insulin, which in turn keeps your blood sugar from shooting sky-high and then crashing down (Raman, 2017).

If you want to be insulin-sensitive, then the type of microbiota you want to have in your gut is called *Coprococcus* (JoJack, 2023). This is because this type of bacteria produces butyrate in your gut. The one you want to avoid having high quantities of, on the other hand, is Flavonicafractor. While the research studying these kinds of bacteria is also in its early stages, they indicate something very interesting: It might be possible to treat insulin resistance and diabetes and even to prevent them by carefully modulating your gut microbiome. For that to be a definitive conclusion, though, a lot of research still needs to be done, especially given the number of microorganisms populating your gut microbiome.

Antibodies Production

We've already established that the gut microbiome contributes to and strengthens your immune system, but how exactly does it do that? To start, let's first understand how the immune system works. Your immune system is made up of something called antibodies. Antibodies are produced by your white blood cells; their job is to attach themselves to viruses, disease-bringing bacteria, and the like and then destroy them. Each white blood cell in your veins carries something called a B receptor (BCR) (Li et al., 2020). The BCR determines what your antibodies can and cannot latch onto. Each BCR is unique, meaning that different kinds of antibodies can attach themselves to different things. On the whole, you want to have diverse antibodies so that you can be protected against all sorts of diseases.

So then, where does your gut microbiome come into this picture? Well, antibodies aren't just produced in your blood. A fair number of them are produced in the mucosal lining of your intestines, where all that microbiota hangs out. Your bloodstream produces two types of antibodies: IgM and IgG. Your intestines produce another type known as IgA, which we mentioned earlier. However, it's not that your intestinal microbes produce these antibodies directly. Rather it's that they synthesize immune tissues, and these antibodies are created just in case any harmful bacteria in the intestines manage to get into your bloodstream because that can happen.

Essentially, your gut microbiota strengthens your immune system by producing additional antibodies that your blood cells can't produce. Not only that, but they prepare them well in advance, before the illness or infection they can attach themselves to even enters your body. Should that illness enter your body, they send those antibodies forth, ensuring you retain your health and strength. Aside from that, your gut microbiome reprograms your white blood cells to create the right antibodies for a disease, further solidifying your immune system's ability to fight it off (University of Bern, 2020).

Antioxidant Production

Another way your gut microbiota helps protect your health and bolster your immune system is by lending a hand with antioxidant production. Antioxidants are a kind of compound that can put an end to free radicals roaming across your body. Free radicals are independent molecules that have been linked to all sorts of disorders like Alzheimer's and cardiovascular diseases and age-related issues like cataracts (Villines, 2017). Simply put, there are things you want to avoid gallivanting around your body and increasing the amount of antioxidants you ingest and produce is the way to go about doing that.

One of the best ways to get more antioxidants into your system is to simply eat foods that have them in high quantities. When antioxidants enter your gut, they have an interesting, two-way interaction with your gut microbiota. The antioxidants in your system improve the health of your gut microbiota, while your gut microbiota increases those antioxidants' capacity. Antioxidants look out for your gut microbiota by encouraging the growth of good bacteria and discouraging the growth of bad ones. The good bacteria then promote antioxidants' capacity by increasing their steady-state plasma levels. This makes them more reactive and, thus, better at doing their jobs (Uchiyama et al., 2022).

Preventing Inflammation

Inflammation is your body's natural response to an irritant of some sort, such as a germ or a foreign object (like something in your eye) entering your system. An inflamed area—be it inside or outside your body—will get red, hot to the touch, and swollen (*National Center for Biotechnology Information*, 2018). This is something that your gut microbiota can also help with. Primarily, they can prevent inflammation in the gut by stimulating certain kinds of cells that can prevent inflammation. In addition, they can keep whatever irritant was trying to cause said irritation from leaking into your bloodstream. Your gut microbiota can do this because they actively regulate your gut's permeability, meaning what gets to leak through to the bloodstream and what doesn't.

When an area of your body gets inflamed, your immune system usually sends something called cytokines to that area, and it's these things that cause the inflammation. Certain substances that your gut microbiome produces can reduce that inflammation. One such substance is short-chain fatty acids, which block the pathways that cytokines usually use to get to the area with the irritant in question and cause it to swell and whatnot (Al Bander et al., 2020). Another anti-inflammatory substance that the gut microbiota produce is butyrate, which actively reduces inflammation when it occurs by similarly blocking the pathways cytokines use.

Aside from cytokines, there's another marker of inflammation known as C-reactive protein (CRP). CRP can also be regulated, thereby causing inflammation to go down when specific microorganisms in the gut produce certain enzymes. These microorganisms are Bifidobacterium and Lactobacillus, which you want to have plenty of in your gut for the reason explained above.

Fermentation

A final benefit that your gut microbiota has to offer you, at least where your metabolism is concerned, is that it can help you digest indigestible carbs by fermenting them. By now, you probably know that eating foods that are rich in dietary fiber is good for you. Unfortunately, the typical Western diet is low in fiber for the most part, even though it's been proven that such a diet can easily lead to inflammatory bowel disease, type 2 diabetes, and other similar metabolic diseases (Cronin et al., 2021). The good news is eating more fiber can reverse these things, and the reason for this is simple: It's because your gut microbiota can kick-start a microbial fermentation process to deal with that fiber and produce short-chain fatty acids as a byproduct.

Those acids, in turn, prevent metabolic diseases and improve your blood sugar levels. As you'll remember, they also prevent inflammation and have the added benefit of preventing all sorts of diseases, disorders, and conditions, such as cardiovascular diseases, certain kinds of cancer, and obesity. When you consider the added benefit of protecting your brain and liver that short-chain fatty acids bring to the table, it makes sense to maintain a diet that promotes a healthy and diverse gut microbiome, don't you think?

Chapter 4:

Gut Microbes Control Your Mind

As you discovered in earlier chapters, your gut microbiome is your second brain and has a very interesting two-way relationship with your actual brain. That means that it affects your brain in some pretty unique ways. As a basic example, your gut microbiome can lift brain fog, which a lot of people experience from time to time, and that can be otherwise hard to resolve. Besides that, your gut microbiota can also influence your cognitive development—at least according to the early studies we have on hand. There's still much to learn and much to be studied where the mind-gut connection is concerned, but what has been uncovered makes it all too clear that a healthy and balanced gut microbiome has many cerebral benefits to offer you.

The Gut-Brain Health

The fact that your gut and your brain can communicate with one another has some very interesting implications for your mental health and the overall well-being of your brain. Your gut microbiome is a very complex environment, as you've learned, and the slightest change in that environment can alter your gut's permeability. This can cause different chemical compounds (which are produced by your gut microbiota) to leak into your bloodstream in various concentrations. Some of these compounds are neuroactive, which means they can directly influence your brain and mental health. This is one reason why your gut microbiota can affect the development of both your central and enteric nervous systems. It's also why it's known to affect several neural conditions, such as neuro-immune mediated disorders, motility disorders, neurodegenerative diseases like Alzheimer's, and behavioral disorders (Strandwitz, 2018).

There are certain bacteria in your gut microbiome that produce a number of neurotransmitters. The most important among these neurotransmitters are serotonin, the happiness hormone; dopamine, which allows you to feel and experience pleasure; norepinephrine, which among other things, controls your stress reactions; and gamma-aminobutyric acid (GABA), which has a calming effect on you. The fact that your gut microbiota can produce more of these substances can dramatically affect your mental health. An imbalance in your gut microbiota, known as dysbiosis, and any inflammation of your gut can have a similar effect. In fact, these two things have been directly linked to various mental health disorders, such as depression and anxiety disorders, through several different studies (Clapp et al., 2017). The good news is that mental health disorders can be treated (or at least alleviated) to some degree by re-establishing balance in your gut microbiome via eating well and taking probiotics. Take depression, for example. Scientists have found that if you're struggling with depression, you're twice as likely to see improvements in your well-being and mood if you were to start taking probiotic supplements (Pinto-Sanchez et al., 2017).

Based on all this, it can be reasonably said that a healthy gut equals a healthy nervous system and a healthy brain. Hence, it also means efficient and balanced brain functioning and performance. One study conducted in 2004 proves as much. This study specifically examined the memory capabilities of mice with healthy gut microbiomes and ones with unhealthy, imbalanced ones. The findings revealed that the first group of mice had higher levels of Brain-Derived Neurotrophic Factors (BDNF) (Arentsen et al., 2015). If you're wondering why that's important, then you should know that high levels of BDNF equal a reduced risk of developing conditions like dementia and Alzheimer's (Bathina & Das, 2015). BDNF is also essential for managing stress and regulating your mood and cognitive functions.

Your gut microbiota can also affect your neurophysiological functions. More specifically, the prevalence of obesity-related microbes in your gut can affect your neurophysiological functions. These, you see, can make your guts more permeable, thereby allowing more chemicals to slip into your bloodstream. Studies show that when you have an abundance of such microbes in your system, you end up with more markers for inflammation and even brain injury, which clearly shows that the state of your gut microbiota can and does affect both your physiological and psychological health (Osadchiy et al., 2019).

Brain Fog

Given the cerebral and cognitive benefits that your gut microbiome can provide, it probably isn't all that surprising to hear that it can help with a little something known as brain fog. Truthfully, brain fog is less a medical condition in and of itself and more a not-so-fun little medical symptom that accompanies other conditions. It can cause many different problems, the most obvious one being a lack of clarity (Higuera, 2022). People with brain fog typically find it hard to think clearly, just like you'd have difficulty seeing clearly if you were walking through an actual fog. Hence the name. It can also cause other problems, such as having trouble remembering things and finding it difficult to concentrate.

Brain fog can be caused by all manner of things, such as stress, sleep deprivation, and the kind of diet you're on. So, it's likely something you've experienced at some point in your life, perhaps while pulling an all-nighter. Knowing that balancing out your gut microbiome can help dispel brain fog can be very helpful to know since you might experience it again sometime in the future too.

Brain fog often occurs when your BDNF levels go down due to one of the reasons above, like stress. The kind of food that you eat plays a crucial role in how much BDNF is produced in your brain. Your brain starts producing less and less BDNF when you eat a diet full of carbs and refined sugar (Molteni et al., 2002). Such a diet also supports the development of potentially harmful microorganisms (Brown et al., 2006). All this results in your brain losing some of its ability to produce BDNF and, thus, create new memories and learn new things. That is the very definition of brain fog.

That's not all though. Your stress levels, a known cause of brain fog, can lead to the very same results. Remember how your gut microbiome creates all these neurotransmitters, like dopamine and norepinephrine? According to studies, chronic stress directly affects your gut microbiome's ability to keep producing them. This is because your gut microbiome is programmed to respond directly to stress. This isn't a problem for fleeting, momentary stress. It is, however, a huge problem where chronic stress is concerned. Continually feeling stressed means your gut's neurotransmitter production is constantly interrupted. That, in turn, means you end up with fewer chemicals that make it possible to think clearly and remember things well.

Cognitive Development

Your cognitive functions mean your ability to learn things, remember them, and use them later in practical ways (Fazzaura Putri et al., 2023). Aside from producing more neurotransmitters that can help with these functions, your gut microbiome can help with your cognitive development. More specifically, having more of certain kinds of microorganisms in your gut microbiome can help with this. Some examples of such microorganisms that immediately come to mind are Bacteroidetes and Lactobacillaceae. When your gut microbiome starts losing one of these microorganisms, then your cognitive development takes a hit. For example, if your Bacteroides levels start decreasing, your hippocampus starts losing its functional and structural plasticity. Similarly, your BDNF levels start going down because that's one of the substances that Bacteroides is in charge of regulating. If, on the other hand, your Lactobacillaceae levels start decreasing, then your gut microbiome starts producing less butyrate. You need your butyrate levels to be high because having low butyrate levels also means being low on BDNF.

Just as there are bacteria that are good for your cognitive development, some are bad for it. One example is Firmicutes, as studies have managed to connect it to neurodegenerative disorders like Alzheimer's. They've also established that Firmicutes interfere with your neurotransmitters' pathways, which is why they're bad for cognitive development. The same kind of observation can be made about other microbiota like Proteobacteria and Actinobacteria. If you want to improve things like your learning abilities and memory, then one thing you need to do is focus on rebalancing your gut microbiota, which you can do either by changing your diet or taking certain probiotics.

Sleep Regulation

There seem to be a great many people around the world who are struggling with sleep. Some aren't able to fall asleep until the late hours of the night and end up sleep-deprived as a result. Others have full-blown insomnia, meaning they have trouble falling or staying asleep and end up incredibly exhausted throughout the day. Many of these people take medication for their various sleep disorders, but they don't realize that they may not have to. Many people could avoid taking medication to manage their sleep disorder by regulating their gut microbiome instead since it also plays an important role in sleep regulation.

Current studies indicate that the microbiota in your gut and the circadian genes are intimately connected. Everyone has an internal clock of some sort that tells you when to wake up within a 24-hour cycle (Rijo-Ferreira & Takahashi, 2019). If you've ever unintentionally woken up five minutes before you had to or when you usually wake up for work on a day off, then you know what I'm talking about. Your internal clock is known as your circadian rhythm, and it's controlled by your circadian genes. Your gut microbiota interacts with these genes to alter your circadian rhythm. The top microbiota that influence these genes are Bacteroidales, Lactobacillales, and Clostridiales, which make up about 60% of your gut microbiome (Li et al., 2018). The way your gut microbiome works makes it anything but static. Instead, it's ever-fluctuating, depending on if it's night or day. If you want to be able to enjoy a good night's sleep, then you want certain kinds of microbiota to be in abundance at certain points of the day and night. If you have an inflammation in your gut, for example, then that inevitably disturbs your microbiota balance, which in turn interferes with your circadian genes and makes it harder for you to sleep. Interestingly, when this happens, the opposite occurs, and your circadian genes interfere with your gut microbiome, making it even more out of balance in the process.

Mood

It's reasonable that your gut microbiota would impact your mood, given how it affects your sleep—no one is exactly cheerful when they don't get enough sleep—and the existence of the gut-brain axis. However, Your gut microbiota can do more than make you a little cranky or moody. An extremely out-of-balance microbiome can rapidly lead to mood disorders, including bipolar disorder and depressive disorder (Huang et al., 2019). These are two conditions that about 10% of the global population is currently struggling with. Researchers have found that individuals struggling with such disorders, particularly stress-related mood disorders like depression, often have thinner mucosal barriers in their guts and an unbalanced gut microbiome.

This makes sense when you remember that an unbalanced gut microbiome equals lower levels of serotonin and dopamine, which are heavily related to how you feel. More than 90% of the serotonin in your body is made in your guts, after all, and people who struggle with depression tend to have very low levels of serotonin. Of course, depression isn't the only mood disorder that can be linked to your gut microbiome. There's also a solid connection between it and bipolar disorder (BD). People with BD are low on certain types of microbiota and have an overabundance of others. If you suffer from BD, which microbiota you have an abundance of depends on whether your symptoms are more manic or depressive. If they're manic, then you'll have too many of two microbiota called Escherichia coli and Bifidobacterium adolescentis. If you're more on the depressive side, then you'll have a lot of Stercoris in your guts. In either case, balancing out your gut microbiota will only help you and your ability to manage your symptoms.

Stress Response

As you may have learned so far, stress can have many different symptoms, but one of the leading ones is stomachaches. Stomachaches can be triggered by your gut microbiome too. Your gut has the enteric nervous system, which is in charge of controlling your general digestive processes. When your gut microbiome changes, even if it's only a slight change, it can impact your enteric nervous system (Appleton, 2018). As a result, your enteric nervous system can send problematic signals to your central nervous system, causing mood disorders and triggering symptoms that are similar to anxiety. Furthermore, these changes can cause irritation and inflammation in your gut, with stomachaches being a common symptom. Those stomachaches can result in your stress response becoming activated. This, right here, is the very reason why gut disorders such as irritable bowel disorder often come hand in hand with stress disorders like anxiety.

On top of that, like your brain, your stress response also has a bilateral relationship with your gut. So, just as your gut can affect your stress levels, your stress levels can affect your gut health. Mainly, stress can make your guts more permeable, which allows more microbiota to cross the gut lining and sneak into your bloodstream (Dinan & Cryan, 2012). This causes the general makeup of your gut microbiome to change, which in turn causes your stress response to become even worse. At the same time, it can worsen other conditions, such as depression, if you also suffer from those. The good news is that existing studies show that this is another issue that can be fixed by simply changing your diet and getting some probiotic help. This is true even in cases where you have conditions like IBD since, in such cases, those probiotics can help fix your gut permeability, along with the makeup of your microbiome.

Brain Aging

Considering the link between your gut microbiome and degenerative conditions like Alzheimer's, the fact that your microbiota can affect how quickly your brain ages makes a lot of sense. Studies have uncovered a definite connection between the changes that your gut microbiome goes through as you age and the degenerative changes that accompany aging. If you want to decrease your chances of experiencing the degenerative and debilitating effects that can come with growing older, then taking care of your gut health is imperative. If your gut microbiome is out of balance, it can cause inflammation in your brain, which can steadily worsen the effects of aging (Alsegiani & Shah, 2022).

The thing about aging is that different parts, organs, and systems of the body age at different rates. Of course, they all "live" for the same amount of time. There's no situation where the heart stops beating two days after the liver stops working or something like that. But your brain may grow old more quickly than your heart, for example, and the same goes for other parts of your body. Maintaining your gut health, including the health and well-being of your gut microbiota, can decrease your chances of this happening. It can ensure that your body ages in an evenly distributed way—if that makes sense. According to one study, your gut microbiota can be used to slow down the rate at which your brain ages and thus improve your cognitive abilities (Boehme et al., 2022).

As you age, your gut microbiome starts losing some of its diversity. This starts happening around your thirties. That doesn't mean things take a turn wholly for the worse. In fact, some studies have found that centenarians have higher levels of certain microbiota that have now become associated with longevity. Still, the fact remains that your microbiome changes as you age, and that change can adversely affect your brain health if you don't manage it well. Your gut microbiota actively contributes to your brain health as you grow older.

Aside from preventing neural inflammation, your gut microbiome can slow neural decline and prevent your neurotransmitter levels from dropping. For instance, a healthy gut microbiome with enough Bacteroides, among other things, can protect your hippocampus from aging and ensure its longevity. This is all thanks to how intimately connected the gut microbiome is to your physical and mental health, as you will discover momentarily.

Chapter 5:

The Link Between Your
Gut and Your Health

All diseases begin in the gut. –**Hippocrates**

As we learned from the last chapter, your gut microbiome can help your brain health and longevity a great deal, as well as look out for your mental well-being. How about your physical health, then? Are there any conditions that your microbiota can help prevent? How about any that they can fight off? As it turns out, there are plenty of both. It has been revealed through numerous studies that your gut microbiota is linked to various immunological and neurological disorders and diseases. You'll learn more about this shortly. Some of these are metabolic disorders, such as diabetes. Others are understandably gut-related, like Inflammatory Bowel Disease (IBD). Some are rather unexpected since you wouldn't really think that there's a connection between your gut and different types of cancer. The health of your gut microbiome is directly related to all these things and more. You can avoid and overcome all of these things if you keep your microbiome well-balanced and strong.

Metabolic Disorders

Your gut microbiome is intimately connected with a whole set of various metabolic disorders. Your metabolism is the process your body uses to convert the food that you eat into energy. Metabolic disorders are disorders that have to do with this process (*Metabolic Disorders*, n.d.). They happen when abnormal chemical reactions occur in your body, disrupting your metabolism. If your metabolism were a machine, a metabolic disorder would occur when something got stuck between its cogs. There are three main metabolic disorders that your gut is connected to. These are

- Diabetes

- Obesity

- Non-alcoholic fatty liver disease

As you probably know, diabetes is a disease that is related to blood sugar levels. In medical terms, your blood sugar is known as your blood glucose. Generally speaking, you want your blood glucose levels to be below a certain point. You want to avoid it being too high or too low. The glucose in your blood is derived from the food you consume. Your cells use this glucose as a source of energy, which is made possible by a hormone called insulin. (*What Is Diabetes?* 2016). Sometimes, however, your body is unable to produce enough insulin or just can't use it as efficiently as it can. When this happens, all or most of that glucose remains in your blood. In other words, it is unable to get into your cells. As a result, your blood sugar level remains high, and this is the very situation known as diabetes.

Diabetes is problematic because it can lead to a wild array of other disorders and diseases over time. For instance, diabetes can easily cause you to experience heart disease, have a stroke, or give you nerve damage. At the same time, it can result in problems with your eyesight, kidney disease, dental issues, and even foot problems. At present, a staggering amount of people have diabetes. One out of ten Americans are diagnosed with diabetes every year, which means that roughly 37 million people are currently living with this disorder (*Type 2 Diabetes*, 2021).

Diabetes has a lot to do with both the food you eat and your gut microbiome, which makes sense given that your gut microbiota comes into direct contact with the food that enters your body. Take type 2 diabetes, for instance, which is the type of diabetes where your body isn't able to make enough insulin. According to one study, there's a kind of reverse relationship between it and the amount of dietary fiber you consume (Li, Stirling, et al., 2020). At the same time, dietary fiber has a parallel relationship with your gut microbiome. This means that the more dietary fiber you have in your diet, the less likely you'll develop Type 2 diabetes and the healthier your gut microbiome will be.

That's not the only connection between diabetes and your gut microbiome. There's also some evidence indicating that there's a link between your gut microbiome and your lipopolysaccharide (LPS) levels. Your LPS levels are regulated by your intestinal microflora. You need this to be the case because when your microflora isn't able to do this, your likelihood of developing diabetes increases. Similarly, evidence shows that people with diabetes have less microbiota in their guts that can produce butyrate. Though the connection between butyrate and diabetes still needs to be explored more, the fact that there is one is pretty clear.

Diabetes is a condition that often goes hand in hand with obesity, which is very closely tied to your diet. With this being the case, it's more than understandable that there would also be a connection between it and your gut microbiome. Obesity can be defined as having excessive fat deposits in your body. Traditionally, medical professionals would judge whether someone is obese or not by looking at their body mass index (BMI). Your BMI is calculated by dividing your weight by your height (*Body Mass Index (BMI)*, 2020). If the resultant figure is over 25, you're considered overweight. If it's over 30, however, then you're considered to be obese (*Obesity*, 2022). Between 2017 and 2020, 41.9% of the US population was diagnosed with obesity, and the situation hasn't improved much since then (*Adult Obesity Facts*, 2021). You can guess just how problematic the general population's diet is and how damaging it can be to their gut microbiome.

Your gut microbiome plays a crucial role in obesity. If it's out of balance and unhealthy, it will certainly contribute to it. Take the right measures to improve it, and you can use your gut microbiota to treat your obesity. This is because your gut microbiota produces all sorts of substances, like enzymes, short-chain fatty acids, and vitamins, that can then enter your bloodstream and impact your metabolic processes (Liu et al., 2021). For this to work in your favor, you need to have a certain amount of the right kinds of microbiota in your gut. That means not having an overabundance of Firmicutes, for example, but having more Bacteroides because if there's one thing studies have shown, it's that obese people have a lot of the former and not enough of the latter. This is why these days, scientists consider your Firmicutes/Bacteroidetes as biomarkers of obesity.

Other kinds of microbiota you may want more of in your system are those belonging to microbiota families like the Lactobacillus and Akkermansia. Several studies have linked these hard-to-produce microbiota groups to weight loss, which is why you want them populating your gut if you're struggling with obesity. While you do want to have plenty of certain kinds of bacteria, you do not want them to be the sole residents of your gut. This is because various other studies have shown that non-obese people have rich and diverse gut microbiomes. Obese people, on the other hand, don't have a great deal of diversity.

One way you can ensure that you have a rich and diverse gut microbiome is to change your diet. Another is to start taking probiotics, which are essentially living bacteria. You can also take prebiotics, which are made from limited digestible foods, and synbiotics, which are a mixture of both limited digestible foods and prebiotics (Davis, 2016). By doing these things, you can actively change your gut's general makeup and composition, thereby warding yourself against obesity.

A final metabolic disorder that your gut microbiome is connected to is a non-alcoholic fatty-liver disease

(NAFLD). NAFLD is a condition where fatty tissue builds up in your liver. Ordinarily, this happens when you drink too much alcohol too often. However, the condition can be caused by other factors too, which is where the "non-alcoholic" part of this disease comes in. Though NAFLD can be harmless, if left unchecked, it can be damaging enough to scar your liver, which is a condition known as cirrhosis. At the same time, NAFLD can lead to other disorders, like diabetes, kidney disease, high blood pressure, and serious liver damage. The most common cause of NAFLD is obesity or being overweight (*Non-Alcoholic Fatty Liver Disease (NAFLD)*, 2017).

The fact that NAFLD is related to weight issues means it's also related to your diet and, thus, your gut microbiota. Your gut microbiota can contribute to NAFLD in several ways. First, your gut microbiota ferments carbs and creates short-chain fatty acids (SCFAs), as you'll recall (Jasirwan et al., 2019). These SCFAs then kick-start the production of an enzyme called DNL in the liver. Meanwhile, it modulates the endocannabinoid system, which plays a part in your eating habits and regulates your ability to metabolize choline, which is a compound that's in charge of transporting lipids (meaning fat) to other parts of the body. When these processes are interrupted, fatty tissue naturally accumulates in your liver. Left unchecked, this starts doing damage to your liver, and if things go on that way for long enough, it can easily result in one of the many health problems we've touched on, including obesity and heart disease.

Inflammatory Bowel Disease (IBD)

Inflammatory Bowel Disease refers to two different conditions: Ulcerative colitis and Crohn's disease. Ulcerative colitis, which is a bit of a mouthful, is a condition that occurs in your large intestine—meaning your colon—and your rectum. It damages these areas and usually starts at the rectum, then spreads higher up to the colon. Crohn's disease, on the other hand, can occur in any part of your intestinal tract, including your mouth. More often than not, though, it afflicts a part of your small intestine and spreads to your large intestine over time. In versions of IBD, the affected area becomes inflamed. Of course, with Crohn's disease, multiple layers of your GI tract can become inflamed, whereas, with Ulcerative colitis, only the outer layer will experience inflammation (*CDC -What Is Inflammatory Bowel Disease (IBD)?* 2018). Regardless of which type of IBD you have, the most likely symptoms you'll experience are:

- abdominal pain

- diarrhea

- blood stool or rectal bleeding

- general fatigue

- weight loss

As for where your gut microbiome comes into the IBD picture, studies show that IBD can be influenced by having abnormal levels of certain types of bacteria in your gut (Kim et al., 2023). It turns out that dysbiosis (an imbalance in your gut microbiome) in your gut can easily lead to both Crohn's disease and ulcerative colitis. Not only that, but any changes to your gut microbiome can trigger either form of IBD too. This is why the makeup of the gut microbiome of a healthy individual is very different from that of someone with IBD. According to the ten or so studies on the matter, people with IBD have abnormally high quantities of 21 different microbiota in their gut. At the same time, they have much lower levels of biodiversity in their gut.

Scientists haven't been able to figure out yet whether issues like IBD result in a gut microbiome imbalance or if it's the other way around. This question is a bit of a "did the chicken come from the egg or the egg from the chicken first?" conundrum, and understandably so. It's also likely that the two conditions can trigger one another, especially given how complex the gut microbiome is and how susceptible to change it is.

One thing that can be concluded from all the existing studies is that a balanced, diverse, and healthy gut microbiome equals the absence of conditions such as IBD. Another thing that can be concluded is that if you do have IBD, you can treat it by changing your diet and taking probiotics since balancing your gut microbiome can soothe this issue (Ries, 2023).

Mental Health Disorders

Thanks to the gut-brain axis and the fact that hormones such as serotonin are produced in the gut, it's by now a well-established fact that your gut can influence your brain. More importantly, it can impact your mind and mental well-being. This means that your gut microbiome can play a significant part in whether you develop certain mental health disorders and conditions or not. So far, the gut microbiome has been linked to four key mental health conditions. These are:

- Alzheimer's disease

- Parkinson's disease

- Autism Spectrum Disorder (ASD)

- Depressive Disorder

Alzheimer's disease is a very common type of dementia. As a progressive degenerative disease, it starts with mild memory loss and can progress to the point that you lose your ability to even hold a conversation. As of 2020, there were about 5.8 million Americans living with Alzheimer's disease; so far, no real cure for it has been found (*What Is Alzheimer's Disease?* 2020). Similarly, the cause of the disease isn't really known either, though the prevalent theory is that it happens because of protein buildup around brain cells, the cause of which is, again, unknown.

Interestingly enough, studies indicate that the cause might be your gut microbiome, or at least that it might be related to it. One study indicated that changes to your gut microbiome might be responsible for Alzheimer's, thanks to the gut-brain axis (Cammann et al., 2023). This study shows that when your gut microbiome becomes less diverse, the speed of the onset of diseases such as Alzheimer's picks up. On the other hand, when you have a diverse gut microbiome, the disease starts progressing slower, assuming you have it. If you don't have it, then you effectively provide yourself with an additional layer of protection against Alzheimer's. Preventing Alzheimer's in this way is a good idea, especially if it runs in your family since it's a genetic condition.

So far, scientists have been able to identify 20 different microbiota that can slow down or prevent the development of Alzheimer's disease. They've also identified various microbiota that inflame the disease if they populate your gut microbiome in large quantities (Varesi et al., 2022). Typically, these microbiota have inflammatory properties. They also seem to be genetically inherited, though their density can be altered through diet and medication. However, the fact that these microbiota can be genetically inherited may not be such a bad thing since they can then be used as biomarkers. Once you spot these biomarkers, you can use them as risk indicators and adjust your diet and medication accordingly. In other words, you can use your gut microbiota as warning signs, so to speak, and then alter your gut microbiome to take preventative measures against Alzheimer's or slow it down.

Then there's Parkinson's disease. Parkinson's disease is a condition where you lose nerve cells in a part of your brain known as substantia nigra (*Parkinson's Disease*, 2022). This causes you to start losing control over your bodily movements. This is why people who have Parkinson's experience twitching limbs almost constantly, along with stiffness, shaking, and trouble maintaining their balance and stability.

As with Alzheimer's, your gut microbiota affects the progression of Parkinson's disease and even your risk of developing it. In fact, your gut microbiota can influence both the severity of Parkinson's disease's symptoms and its progression. One indicator of the strong connection between your gut microbiome and Parkinson's is that people with the condition often experience gastrointestinal issues before the official Parkinson's symptoms begin. The change within your gut microbiome that most dramatically affects Parkinson's has to do with microbiota that can produce short-chain fatty acids (SCFAs). When dysbiosis occurs in the microbiome, and the amount of microbiota that can create SCFAs decreases, your risk of developing Parkison's increases. Likewise, the progression of the disease, if you have it, speeds up. The same thing happens when the quantity of pro-inflammatory microbiota increases in your gut (Romano et al., 2021).

Another way in which your gut microbiome may contribute to Parkinson's has to do with its ability to produce ghrelin. Ghrelin is a neuropeptide (a chemical messenger made up of small-chain amino acids) with neuroprotective properties and can stimulate your appetite (Bayliss & Andrews, 2013). Studies show that people who have Parkinson's have much lower ghrelin levels than people who don't. Therefore, having high levels of ghrelin is vital to protect your brain against diseases like Parkinson's. The only way to ensure that that's the case is to have a well-balanced and healthy gut microbiome. This is because your gut microbiome is responsible for regulating how ghrelin is expressed throughout your body. If your microbiome is thrown off balance, you cannot produce all the ghrelin you need (Leeuwendaal et al., 2021). You will also become unable to use the ghrelin you already have effectively, which makes you more susceptible to Parkinson's disease.

As surprising as this might be to hear, your gut microbiome plays a pivotal role in Autism Spectrum Disorder (ASD) as well. Studies have revealed that the gut microbiome of children with ASD is vastly different from that of neurotypical children, meaning children without such disorders. They have higher quantities of certain microbiota and lower quantities of others (Taniya et al., 2022). This starts making a lot of sense when you factor in how many people with ASD experience various kinds of gastrointestinal issues.

One very interesting finding from a study was that giving antibiotics to young kids can significantly affect the progression of ASD at the onset of the disorder. Meanwhile, the presence of microbiota that can produce SCFAs in your gut microbiome can influence the development of ASD. How you were born can determine whether you have enough of these helpful bacteria in your gut. Studies have found that children born via natural birth have more of these good microbiota in their guts than children born via c-section. This is because more of the mother's microbiota is transferred to their children during natural birth.

Of course, not all maternal microbiota are good for the baby, which is one reason why birth mothers need to be careful what they eat when carrying and delivering their children. One example of such a microbiota is called IL-17a. Researchers have found that children become more prone to displaying autism-like symptoms when their birth mothers have high levels of IL-17a in their system. Of course, IL-17a isn't the only microbiota to impact children and whether they will have autism or not. There are potentially many other microbiota that do the same (Orenstein, 2021). However, What these microbiota are isn't well known yet, since scientists have only recently begun looking into the connection between the gut microbiome and ASD.

All that being said, it's important to note that while people with ASD have specific microbiota concentrations, there doesn't seem to be any one kind of microbiota that "causes" ASD. At least, there don't seem to be any that can be found. It's more plausible that your microbiome simply encourages and drives ASD symptoms rather than acts as its root cause. It's also plausible that these symptoms can be better managed and somewhat alleviated through targeted microbiome treatments. A study, which was conducted in the year 2000, shows as much. This study effectively proved that certain microbiota can improve both the speech and social skills of children with autism eight out of ten times (Sandler et al., 2000). So, as long as the children in question took the probiotics prescribed to them, they observed remarkable progress in these areas. Though their symptoms didn't just up and vanish, the probiotic help made their lives much easier.

A similar thing happened in a study from 2017 when children with ASD underwent a microbiota transplant. The microbiota that were introduced to their system were given to them by donors who didn't have ASD. Soon after, not only did the participants of the study experience improvements in their ASD-related symptoms, but the gastrointestinal issues they'd been wrestling with for years were alleviated as well (Kang et al., 2019). If all this doesn't prove that there's a link between your gut microbiota and ASD, then I'm not sure what will. However, how far that link goes is still up for debate, and only more research can reveal the truth of this matter.

A final mental health disorder that your gut microbiome seems to be connected to is major depressive disorder. Major depressive disorder is an exhausting and debilitating condition, to say the least. People with major depressive disorder deal with a near-constant depressive mood—obviously—as well as general fatigue, appetite issues, and insomnia. As of 2020, it's estimated that a total of 21 million people have major depressive disorder, and that's just in the US (*Major Depression*, 2022). More often than not, major depressive disorder is treated with a mix of antidepressants and therapy. Sadly, statistics show that this combination doesn't really work for 10-30% of people who try it. The good news here is that for these people, the connection between the gut microbiome and major depressive disorder can become a solution if it's used right.

The link between depression and the gut microbiome is easier to track than most mental health disorders. There's the fact that serotonin is produced in the gut, for example. Another sign is how stress can cause dysbiosis in the gut, thereby messing with the gut microbiome and causing the gut to "leak" toxic microbiota that ultimately make their way to the brain, where they wreak havoc. As you've already seen in our explorations of the gut-brain axis, your gut microbiota can easily trigger or worsen depressive symptoms. That's not all they can do, though. Some microbiota, for example, can predict depressive symptoms. In fact, there are 16 different microbiota that can do this. If these microbiota are hanging out in your guts in large numbers, then odds are you have (or will soon) started exhibiting depressive symptoms. Some of these microbiota are also found in large quantities in obese people and people with traumatic brain injuries, by the way, which only confirms the bond between these seemingly separate conditions (Radjabzadeh et al., 2022).

As for whether any specific gut microbiota can cause depression... This is a rather tricky question to answer because there are way too many factors to consider where depression is concerned. Still, one study found that a bacteria going by the thankfully pronounceable name Eggerthella seem to overpopulate depressed individuals' guts. Hence, this may be one of the potential causes of major depressive disorder or, at the very least, a contributing factor to it. As before, however, only time will tell whether this is absolutely true or not.

Cardiovascular Disease (CVD)

It should be no surprise that what you eat directly affects your heart health, seeing as it influences things like your blood sugar and blood pressure. It might be a little surprising to hear that your gut microbiome also affects your heart health, at least until you remember how it can influence things like your blood sugar. It's not by chance that the connection between your gut microbiome and metabolic diseases like diabetes exists. The most common cardiovascular disease around the globe is coronary artery disease (CAD), so much so that it is one of the leading causes of mortality in the world. More often than not, CAD is caused by high cholesterol levels, and it has a very intimate relationship with your gut microbiome (Kazemian et al., 2020). This is because your gut microbiota directly influence your cholesterol levels. Your cholesterol levels are partly regulated by your gut lumen (a sort of tubular part of your gut), which helps with cholesterol absorption. Once cholesterol has been absorbed, your liver kicks into gear and metabolizes cholesterol into bile acid, which is then used to help you digest food, among other things.

Naturally, this only happens as it should if you have a healthy and balanced microbiome. If your gut microbiome is unbalanced, though, then the "bad" microbiota in your system renders it less absorbable. As a result, your cholesterol levels remain higher than they should be, and you end up producing less bile acid than you need to. This, in turn, leads to digestion issues as well, which only worsens the situation at hand. Meanwhile, your high cholesterol starts building up in your veins, preventing them from pumping the needed amount of blood to your heart. Deprived of the blood, oxygen, and nutrients it needs, your heart starts weakening, and you eventually end up with coronary artery disease.

CAD isn't the only cardiovascular disease that can be caused by an unhealthy gut microbiome. Similarly, it's not just your gut microbiome that can affect your heart health. Your heart health can also affect your gut microbiome. This is because people who have heart troubles often struggle with other conditions like obesity, which can disrupt the balance of your gut microbiome and cause it to grow less diverse and harmonious (Novakovic et al., 2020). When such dysbiosis occurs in the gut microbiome, your guts sadly become inflamed, which reduces the integrity of your gut barrier and, yet again, causes different microbiota and metabolites to leak out. Among the metabolites that can leak out in this process are short-chain fatty acids and trimethylamine-N-oxide, which scientists believe exacerbate various cardiovascular diseases. While all this is happening, gut microbiome dysbiosis also disrupts the metabolization process of lipids and carbs. This leads to more fats being stored in your body, more cholesterol accumulating in your arteries, and your blood sugar levels rising and remaining high. All of these things contribute to further heart diseases and problems if they go on for long enough.

Human Immunodeficiency Virus (HIV)

The human gut microbiome has become linked to the human immunodeficiency virus (HIV) too. Once you consider how deeply entrenched the gut microbiome is with your immune system, it's easy to see where this connection comes from. HIV, after all, is a disease that attacks your immune system, and its job will only be made easier if your immune system is already weak.

Scientists following along this chain of thought have uncovered some interesting facts about HIV and the gut microbiome. For starters, they've found that the state of your gut microbiome plays a crucial role in how at-risk you are of suffering from an HIV infection (Jennifer A. Fulcher et al., 2022). These scientists have discovered that the kind of bacteria you have in your gut can deter or encourage HIV transmission. As an extension of that, they can be used as a way to both prevent and treat HIV.

Another thing scientists have discovered is that there's a discernible link between your gut microbiome and chronic HIV, which is the second stage of the disease where the virus is multiplying in your body but isn't causing any symptoms yet (*The Stages of HIV Infection*, 2021). This link between your gut microbiome and chronic HIV has allowed scientists to uncover the fact that people who catch HIV usually have decreased levels of certain Bacteroides species in their gut microbiomes. Bacteroides are a kind of bacteria (if you didn't already guess from the name) that ordinarily like hanging out in your lower intestines (Salas & Chang, 2014). Similarly, they've found that people who catch HIV have higher levels of Megasphaera elsdenii. While this microbiota's role in the gut microbiome is as yet unknown, the fact that people with HIV have an abundance of them is troubling. At the very least, it means that this microbiota is something to be explored further, especially as part of further research on HIV treatments and medication.

Cancer

The final health issue that your gut microbiome seems to be connected to is cancer, which is a pretty big issue no matter how you look at it. Studies show that the state of your gut microbiome can impact not only whether or not you develop some type of cancer but also how effective the medication you're given as part of your treatment will be (Cheng et al., 2020). When certain bacteria start overpopulating your gut microbiome, your cancer risk increases (Sadrekarimi et al., 2022). Not only that, but the state of your microbiome directly affects cancer development. For example, let's say that you have a tumor. Scientists have determined that the state and health of your gut microflora can slow down or speed up that tumor's growth. They can do this indirectly by causing inflammation in the guts, which results in certain toxins leaking into your system. These toxins then "feed" the tumor and hasten its growth.

Typically, your immune system would respond to the growth of a tumor and try to do away with it. However, when dysbiosis occurs in your gut microbiome, certain kinds of microbiota actively suppress your immune system, making it much less effective than it could be. As a result, your immune system becomes unable to stop the tumor's growth or slow it down by any real measure. So, the tumor keeps growing and potentially turns into full-blown cancer if it's not caught on time. Today, there are several treatment measures that you could explore should such a thing happen, depending on the severity of your cancer. However, your gut microbiome will affect how effective those treatment methods are, as you know. Studies have found that certain gut microbiota actually increase your resistance to chemo drugs (Cheng et al., 2020). This is problematic because the less resistant you are to chemotherapy, the more easily your cancer can be killed off.

Luckily, this situation can be amended. All you have to do is take some very specific probiotic supplements, which will restore your chemo resistance levels (as in lower them) to what they should be. This will allow the drugs you're taking to work as they should, thereby significantly increasing your chances of beating cancer. This finding has spurred scientists to investigate the gut microbiome-cancer link even more closely. After all, if your gut microbiota can be used to make chemo medications more effective, couldn't they also be used to "treat" cancer? Could the solution to the cancer problem be found in your microbiome? Time will tell... In the meantime, you can always focus on improving the diversity of your gut microbiome, which you'll discover how to do in the next chapter by making sure you have a healthy gut that can offer you all these various benefits we're about to talk about.

Chapter 6:
Improving the Diversity of
Gut Microbiome

The road to health is paved with good intestines!
–Sherry A. Rogers

Now that you've discovered the many, many ways in which your gut microbiome can affect your physical and mental health, one thing should be clear: If you want to lead a healthy and happy life, you need to make sure you have a healthy, well-balanced gut microbiome. Only then can you decrease your risk of hereditary diseases like Alzheimer's and be certain that you avoid other health issues, such as cardiovascular disease, obesity, and major depressive disorder. The simple question you need to ask yourself is, "What do I need to do to ensure my gut microbiome is healthy and well-balanced?" However, the answer is quite lengthy because several factors influence your gut health. For instance, There are probiotics and prebiotics to consider. Then there are fermented foods, polyphenols, and omega-3 fatty acids. There's also the question of which foods to eat and which to avoid. The good news is that you don't have to go on a quest across the internet to discover the secrets of a healthy gut. All you have to do is keep reading.

What Does a Gut-Healthy Diet Entail?

There are many different things you need to eat and consume on a pretty regular basis to make sure you maintain your gut health. These are:

- Certain probiotics

- Certain prebiotics

- Fermented foods

- Fruits and vegetables

- Beans and legumes

- Whole grains (if you can)

Let's start by looking at probiotics, which we have mentioned a couple of times throughout this book. By now, I'm sure you're wondering; what exactly are they? Probiotics are supplements you can take that are partly made of beneficial live bacteria and partly made up of the kinds of yeast that naturally live inside your body (*Probiotics: What Is It, Benefits, Side Effects, Food & Types*, 2020). Probiotics are good for making sure your microbiome remains healthy and balanced and restoring that balance once it's disrupted. That means that they can increase the number of "good" microbiota in your gut when they go down and decrease the levels of "bad" bacteria when they rise. Depending on what kinds of probiotics you're taking, you may enjoy some of the additional benefits they have to offer. Some examples of these benefits could be:

- Helping your gut create more vitamins and enzymes that are essential for your well-being.

- Making your gut walls less leaky, thereby preventing "bad" bacteria from entering your bloodstream.

- Assisting in the digestion of the food you consume.

- Breaking down and absorbing any medication you might be taking.

Now, there are numerous kinds of probiotics you can take. The most common ones fall into one of two categories: Lactobacillus, commonly referred to as L., and Bifidobacteria, which is commonly referred to as B. (Hecht, 2022). L. is a kind of bacteria that produces an enzyme called lactase. As you may have surmised from its name, lactase is used to break down lactose, otherwise known as "milk sugar." I'm sure you've heard of lactose intolerance before. Some people are lactose intolerant because they don't have enough lactase in their system. This can happen if you don't have enough bacteria from the Lactobacillus in your guts, which can and will lead to you being unable to digest milk.

Another thing L. is good for is producing lactic acid, which serves various important functions, such as helping your cells to breathe and aiding your body in the production of glucose (Rush & Barrell, 2021). When you don't have enough L. bacteria in your guts, your lactic acid levels go down, and these processes are disrupted. Your energy levels go down because lactic acid is your muscles' main fuel source. At the same, your health declines since L. further helps you by keeping the number of bad bacteria in your guts low and increases your body's ability to absorb the various minerals that come with the food you eat.

Then there's B., which is the genus of bacteria that are typically used in probiotic supplements. It's also the one found most often in the food you eat. Most probiotic supplements feature B. because they're known to reduce the bad bacteria levels in your gut microbiome. Furthermore, they have a reputation for boosting your immune system and, like L., helping you break down and digest the lactose you ingest.

You can tell which category a certain probiotic fits into by looking at the letter in front of it. If a probiotic supplement reads "B. *something-or-other*," it belongs in the Bifidobacteria genus. If, on the hand, it reads "L. *something-or-other*," then it's from the Lactobacillus genus. Within these different categories, there are a *lot* of probiotics you can take. Obviously, you should always consult your doctor before taking a probiotic, especially if you want to take them to treat a specific problem, like diarrhea or digestion issues, for example. However, knowing what kinds of probiotics are out there and what they're good for can make that conversation much faster. That being said, here are some examples of the most common and popular probiotics you could try:

- *L. acidophilus*: This microbiota is normally found in the small intestines. They can be taken as probiotics and found in certain foods such as yogurt, fermented foods, and soy products (Gao et al., 2022). Studies have shown that it can reduce your risk of developing cardiovascular diseases, improve your heart health if you do have such a disease, prevent and treat certain types of cancer, boost your immunity, and help fix any gastrointestinal problems or diseases you may be struggling with.

- *L. reuteri:* This can be found in your mouth and intestines. According to one study, the ones in your mouth actually help decrease the number of bad bacteria found there, thereby protecting your teeth from cavities (Nikawa et al., 2004). Like most L. bacteria, it helps you to produce lactose. Aside from that, it also aids in digestion and helps you absorb the nutrients you consume. Doctors have discovered many uses for L. reuteri. For instance, it's a recommended treatment method for diabetes, canker sores, high cholesterol, and eczema. Some studies indicate that it may even be a good supplement to take if you have COVID-19 (*Limosilactobacillus Reuteri: Overview, Uses,* n.d.). When you consider that L. reuteri can help quell diarrhea, constipation, and other similar conditions, it becomes clear to see how useful a supplement it can be. L. reuteri can naturally be found in fermented foods like yogurt.

- *B. lactis*: This probiotic is derived from milk and is good for all sorts of things, from helping with food digestion to the absorption of nutrients during that process and even fighting off the bad bacteria in your gut. Ordinarily, it's found naturally in the gut. Like L. reuteri, it can be used to treat any number of conditions, such as diarrhea, constipation, colic, IBD, and even respiratory tract infections. It's known to be a good treatment for cavities and—believe it or not—even hay fever. It might also be good for COVID-19 (*Bifidobacterium Animalis Subsp. Lactis: Overview, Uses, Side Effects*, n.d.).

- *B. animalis*: This is another bacterium that can be found in large quantities in your gut, assuming your gut microbiome is healthy. The aforementioned B. lactis is a subspecies of B. animalis, which can treat and prevent acute diarrhea (especially when it's antibiotic-related) and help with constipation and digestion. At the same time, it can reduce cold and flu symptoms, grant you protection against certain infections like E. coli, and actively support infant growth (Novkovic, 2019).

- *B. breve*: A natural occupant of your intestinal tract, B. breve is great for fending off the kinds of bacteria that can cause various infections in your body. This substance is effective against yeast infections and produces acetic and lactic acid. It is commonly found in breast milk(*Bifidobacterium Breve: Overview, Uses*, n.d.).

As you can see, probiotic supplements are very good for your gut microbiome and health. Hence, they should be made a part of your regular diet. To that end, you can and should take probiotic supplements. Those supplements, however, aren't the only way to introduce the right probiotics to your gut microbiome. A lot of them also exist in numerous different foods. This means you can consume those probiotics naturally by making certain foods a regular part of your diet, as you'll see momentarily. Before we dive into that, however, you have to go over one other kind of supplement you could be taking—prebiotics.

Prebiotics are the food sources that the microbiota in your gut consume to sustain themselves (Cresci, 2022). We all have to eat something, after all. If you have a healthy gut microbiome and are eating the right kinds of food—more on that later—then the prebiotics that exists in the food you consume will make it all the way down to your colon. Here, your microbiota will consume (that's to say, ferment) and metabolize these prebiotics. All sorts of enzymes and chemicals, which you've learned are very good for you, will be created in the process. For example, those short-chain fatty acids we discussed before are created while your microbiota are eating up their prebiotics.

As with probiotics, there are different kinds of prebiotics you could be taking. These different kinds of prebiotics can help you in an array of ways, such as by helping with digestion, creating the neurotransmitters you need to keep your mood elevated, boosting your immune system, suppressing your appetite, getting your bones to absorb more calcium and phosphorus, and thereby making them stronger, and more. Overall, prebiotics fit into one of six categories. These are

- Galacto-oligosaccharides (GOS)

- Hemicellulose-derived oligosaccharides (HDOs)

- Fructans

- Glucose and starch-derived oligosaccharides

- Non-carbohydrate oligosaccharides

- Pectin oligosaccharides (POS)

Galacto-oligosaccharides (GOS) are the primary food source of Bifidobacteria and Lactobacilli, though other types of microbiota (like Firmicutes) enjoy them as well (*Galacto-Oligosaccharides (GOS): Overview, Uses,* n.d.). Taking GOS can help you deal with food allergies, constipation, and eczema. They are most often found in beans, some root vegetables, and dairy products.

Then there are Hemicellulose-derived oligosaccharides (HDOs). HDOs are really effective in reducing bad bacteria populations and inflammation in your gut, as well as producing useful things like butyrate and short-chain fatty acids (Jana et al., 2021). As for Fructans, they improve your blood sugar and triglyceride levels, along with your immune system and overall metabolism (Chong, 2019). They promote the growth of many different kinds of microbiota.

Meanwhile, Glucose and starch-derived oligosaccharides are found in fiber-rich foods, which are great for you. These prebiotics decrease your risk of developing chronic health disorders, such as heart conditions and metabolic conditions like diabetes, and even prevent certain types of cancer because of the kinds of microbiota they support (Adam-Perrot et al., 2009). On the other hand, non-carbohydrate oligosaccharides come from complex carbs like whole grains and are the main food source of anaerobic bacteria (Roberfroid, 1997). They help with digestion, keep the acidity levels of your colon within normal ranges, and prevent gastrointestinal issues.

Lastly, there are Pectin oligosaccharides (POS), which are obviously found in food that's rich in pectin. They make the good bacteria in your gut even better at producing the enzymes you need and promote the growth of both L. and B. microbiota in the colon. Constipation relief, reducing your risk of developing colonic cancer, helping with mineral absorption, and regulating your immune system are only some of its benefits (Wongkaew et al., 2022).

To that end, there are specific kinds of foods that have to be made a part of your everyday diet. These are

- fermented foods

- fruits and vegetables

- beans and legumes

- whole grains (if you can eat them)

The first kind of food that you need to start eating more of is the fermented kind. Fermented foods are food items that have gone through the fermentation process, which encourages the growth of bacteria that are good for you. This automatically makes them rich in probiotics, which means you really can't go wrong with them. The best fermented foods to eat more of for the sake of your gut microbiome are yogurt, sauerkraut, kefir, kimchi, and miso (Rapson, 2018).

Fermented foods have many benefits due to their high probiotic content. For instance, they're known to reduce your risk of developing heart conditions, diabetes, high blood pressure, and inflammation. They improve your general mood and make it easier for you to manage your weight. On a microbial level, fermented foods help your microbiota produce bioactive peptides. These are very useful for you because they're anti-inflammatory, anti-cancer, antioxidative, and anti-many other things that you want to avoid (Akbarian et al., 2022). On top of that, they also help your microbiome make various vitamins too.

Take yogurt, for example. Yogurt is one of the most probiotic-rich things you can ever eat (Palsdottir, 2018). It's absolutely brimming with different kinds of bifidobacteria and lactic acid bacteria. As such, it's great for increasing the diversity of your gut microbiome. Individuals who eat more yogurt have larger amounts of B. animalis in their gut microbiome, among other microbiota, which is great for reducing gut inflammation (Francqueville, 2022). Other benefits that yogurt offer as a result of this are that it increases your bone strength, lowers your blood pressure, reduces diarrhea (especially when it's caused by antibiotics), and even makes managing your weight easier to do. Interestingly enough, yogurt is something that a lactose-intolerant person can freely enjoy. This is because the bacteria in yogurt (which is a kind of bacteria that lactose intolerant people lack) automatically gets to work, turning lactose into lactic acid.

All that being said, it should be noted that not all types of yogurt have probiotics in them. As such, you must pay attention to what kind of yogurt you eat. As a rule, you want to go with yogurt that has either live or active cultures because those labels mean that the bacteria in them are alive and haven't been killed off in the fermentation process (Palsdottir, 2018). The same thing holds true for some kinds of cheeses. Cheeses that are labeled to have "active" or "live" cultures have the kind of bacteria you want to eat and can therefore be consumed without any guilt, although it's probably best to eat them in moderation. Among these cheeses are mozzarella, gouda, cottage cheese, and cheddar—all typical favorites. Aside from being home to good bacteria, such cheeses possess nutrients that are very good for you in general, like selenium, vitamin B12, and calcium.

Sauerkraut is another fermented food you should enjoy. For those of you that don't know, sauerkraut is shredded cabbage fermented in lactic acid bacteria. Yum! It's often used as a topping for hot dogs or plain sausages and tastes rather sour. Sauerkraut is home to lots of immune-boosting probiotics that also serve to keep your gut lining healthy. This makes your gut less "leaky," as you'll recall. Sauerkraut probiotics further support the production of antibodies in your body, reducing your risk of developing inflammation or an infection such as the common cold. These probiotics improve your digestion, restore the bacterial balance in your gut after you finish taking antibiotics, and even help with symptoms of health-related issues like Crohn's disease (Petre, 2020).

An additional fermented food is kefir, which is admittedly an acquired taste. Kefir can be defined as a kind of milk drink that obviously undergoes the fermentation process. Interestingly enough, kefir can be considered a more potent probiotic than yogurt because it's home to 61 different bacterial strains (Bourrie et al., 2016). In fact, there's a probiotic known as L. kefiri, which—as per the name—can only be found in kefir. L. kefiri can prevent the growth of some very harmful bacteria like E. coli in your gut, and it can also protect you from developing cancer (Leech, 2018).

Kefir is an inherently different food from kimchi, which is a kind of spicy Korean dish that's typically made from cabbage. However, the two have one major thing in common; both foods have probiotics that can't be found anywhere else. Kefir has L. kefiri, as you know, while kimchi has the creatively-named L. kimchii (Park et al., 2014). However, L. kimchii isn't the only probiotic in kimchi. The dish is home to many probiotics that help you break down sugar into lactic acid, treat conditions like diarrhea, and both prevent and treat several different issues, such as heart disease, the common cold, some skin conditions, and certain types of cancer (Snyder, 2021). At the same time, they reduce inflammation, slow down the aging process, and, like most probiotics, strengthen your immune system.

The last kind of fermented food I suggest you try out is miso. Miso is a kind of Japanese seasoning that is made by mixing soybeans with a couple of different things—like barley, for instance. Served in paste form, it's an excellent source of fiber and proteins and is chock full of probiotics. The star among these is one that's called *A. oryzae*, which is known to reduce and alleviate gastrointestinal problems such as IBD (Okada et al., 2016). An added benefit of miso is that it doesn't have a lot of antinutrients in it. Antinutrients are compounds found in food products such as soybeans that can attach themselves to the nutrients in your gut, thereby preventing them from being absorbed into your body. The fermentation process that miso undergoes does away with such antinutrients, making miso much easier to digest than some foods. Miso also reduces your risk of developing certain cancers, including stomach cancer, and lessens the cancer-supporting properties that usually come with salty food (Petre, 2017).

Fermented foods like yogurt and miso are beneficial for your gut microbiome and general health. They're not the only food group to possess all these really useful probiotics, though. Fruits and vegetables are very rich in both probiotics and prebiotics as well. As a general rule, if you want to have a diverse gut microbiome, you need to have a green diet. Consider your average, medium-sized apple. It turns out that this single apple contains approximately 100 million bacteria (Lillo-Pérez et al., 2021). That's after said apple has been washed and peeled because most of those bacteria reside in its flesh, not its skin, and even in its core.

If this is true for a simple apple, imagine how many different kinds of bacteria you must be introducing to your guts by simply eating a large variety of fruits and vegetables. Most of these bacteria are good for you, at the very least, since they increase the diversity of your gut microbiome. Of course, different kinds of fruits and vegetables host different kinds of probiotics. So, which fruits and vegetables should you eat a lot of to get the most benefits? Well, you should try to keep things as diversified as possible in this regard, but you shouldn't skip out on the following food products: (Cadman, 2018)

- **Garlic**: The probiotics in it support the growth of healthy bacteria and prevent the growth of bad ones.

- **Onions and their ilk**: This vegetable contains the kind of probiotics that help with digestion and are filled with antioxidants.

- **Leeks**: As members of the onions clan, they also have a high probiotic makeup.

- **Bananas**: This fruit is rich in both probiotics and fiber, meaning it is, therefore, able to promote the growth of good bacteria and prevent things like bloating.

- **Watermelons**: Another fruit that is very rich in prebiotics and also high in vitamin and water content.

- **Grapefruits**: This citrus fruit is similarly rich in fiber, prebiotics, and vitamins C and A.

If vegetables and fruits are an essential part of your diet for the sake of your gut health, then so are legumes. Legumes can be defined as the seeds or fruits of certain kinds of plants. Some of the most probiotic legumes you can eat are chickpeas, beans of any kind, and lentils. Chickpeas have a lot of prebiotics, as well as probiotics and fiber. They're especially rich in a fiber called raffinose, which, coupled with prebiotics and probiotics, make them especially good for digestion (Nelson, 2022). This is why eating more chickpeas can make bowel movements a lot easier and more regular. It's also why chickpeas can lower your cholesterol and blood sugar levels, prevent certain cancers, and strengthen your bones.

Beans, meanwhile, are known for their ability to increase and strengthen the good microbiota in your gut. Beans mostly have prebiotics, and their oligosaccharide content is especially high, no matter what type of bean you have. Oligosaccharide is a prebiotic that the bacteria in your large intestines love devouring. Actually, their feasting on this prebiotic is the very reason why beans make you gassy. Said gas ends up being a side product of the fermentation that takes place when your microbiota releases enzymes to break down the oligosaccharide in your intestines (Tresca, 2021).

Then there are lentils, which are also rich in prebiotics. The primary type of prebiotics they contain are of the carbohydrate variety, which are fermented by the microbiota in your colon. These prebiotics then help you to transport carbs across your body and store them. The fact that lentils are rich in protein and various micronutrients only adds to their many benefits (Johnson et al., 2020).

Whole grains are a final food group that needs to be made a part of your diet. We're used to thinking of carbs as "the bad guys," but that's not necessarily true, at least not as long as you eat the right kinds of carbs. And by the right kind of carbs, I mean whole grains such as wheat, which are vital for a healthy and well-balanced gut microbiome. This is because whole grains have a great deal of prebiotics to offer you, and this includes fiber, which you know is vital for your gut (*Gut Health*, n.d.). The first thing your gut microbiota will do when you give them whole grains is to metabolize the fiber in them to create those infamous short-chain fatty acids. These will then be used to reduce the acidity levels of your gut, thereby creating the perfect living environment for your gut microbiota. They'll further help you absorb more minerals into your system, improve your gut lining, and provide your gut microbiota with greater energy. In addition, the prebiotics in whole grains will help prevent certain cancers like those of the colon, treat conditions such as IBD, and strengthen your immune system.

There you have it then. If you want to ensure the health of your gut microbiome and, thus, your long-term health and well-being, then you have to eat a varied diet made up of fermented foods, vegetables, fruits, legumes, and whole grains. Your diet cannot consist of just these things, though, as useful as they might be. This is because while these foods are very healthy for you, they lack certain essential nutrients that can be found in different food groups. Because your gut microbiome needs those nutrients to be able to function properly, you need to factor them into your diet too.

Food for Thought

A healthy and diverse gut microbiome needs several kinds of nutrients. One of these nutrients is polyphenols. Polyphenols are a kind of micronutrient that's found in plant-based foods. They have antioxidant properties and can therefore reduce the number of free radicals roaming across your body, mitigating any damage they might do (Wang et al., 2022). Antioxidants are needed to deal with free radicals because they "donate" electrons to free radicals, making them less reactive to the other molecules and compounds around. Meanwhile, antioxidants remain stable even after making that donation.

Polyphenols have an exceptionally high antioxidant content, so much so that few other micronutrients can compete with them in this regard. Of course, there are many different types of polyphenols. Two of the most important ones are flavonoids and phenolic acids. Most healthcare professionals recommend consuming about a gram of these two polyphenols daily. Flavonoids are most commonly found in fruits and vegetables, but things like tea, chocolate, and red wine also have high flavonoid content (Watson, 2019). Since scientists apparently like categorizing and labeling things, flavonoids can be divided into six different sub-categories in and of themselves. These categories are:

- **Anthocyanins**: This flavonoid can be described as a kind of pigment that gives flowers their distinct red or purple color. Hence, they're often found in berries and grapes and therefore exist in large quantities in wine.

- **Isoflavones**: Commonly found in various legumes, soy, and soy products. They're very good at keeping your hormones in balance.

- **Flavones**: These can be defined as the pigments of white and blue flowered plants and help keep inflammation down throughout your body. Foods like parsley, celery, peppermint, and red peppers are rich in them.

- **Flavanones**: Most often found in citrus fruits such as lemons, oranges, and grapefruits. Like flavones, they help keep inflammation down and manage your cholesterol levels.

- **Flavan-3-ols**: An incredibly rich type of flavonoid. Apples, various kinds of teas, strawberries, blueberries, and cocoa have them in abundance.

- **Flavanols**: The kind of flavonoid that's richest in antioxidants. Known to help with cardiovascular diseases, they can be found in various vegetables and fruits—from onions and kale to peaches and berries.

All of these flavonoid types are very good for your gut microbiome health. This is because of several reasons. For one, flavonoids are typically metabolized by your gut microbiota. This results in the production of certain enzymes and metabolites that improves your gut's immune capabilities. At the same time, the antioxidant properties of flavonoids can prevent gastrointestinal inflammation from taking place, which could cause you a whole host of health issues if you let it (Pei et al., 2020).

Another key polyphenol your gut microbiome needs is phenolic acids. Phenolic acids are mostly found in plant-based foods, spices such as anise and cumin, coffee, and fruits like blueberries and plums. They've even been found in cereals, though it's probably a good idea to avoid brands of cereal that are chock-full of sugar if you can. The good thing about phenolic acids is that they can bind polysaccharides like starch, which makes digestion far easier. Some phenolic acids affect certain enzymes that are produced in the gut. These enzymes deal directly with the synthesis of compounds that could otherwise lead to inflammation. This is why phenolic acids are able to keep your inflammation levels down (Kasprzak-Drozd et al., 2021).

When considering polyphenols in general, it's easy to see just how much they can help promote your gut health. For example, the fact that polyphenols have antioxidant properties means they can reduce the effects of aging, particularly degenerative ones. At the same time, they can lower your risk of developing certain kinds of heart disease, and lower your blood sugar and bad cholesterol, thus reducing your risk of developing diabetes. Flavonoids are known to be particularly effective in this regard, which is why scientists are actively exploring them to treat diabetes. After all, flavonoids not only lower your blood sugar levels, but they improve your ability to metabolize fats as well. In recent studies, scientists have discovered that flavonoids reduce your chances of developing type 2 diabetes when they're consumed regularly (Xu et al., 2018).

One other thing that polyphenols are great at preventing is cancer, which is thanks to their anti-inflammatory and antioxidant properties (Kasprzak-Drozd et al., 2021). You see, polyphenols play an active part in managing the biological process that takes place when a tumor initially begins forming. Simply put, they're capable of stopping that process and preventing a tumor from ever forming in the first place. They can do this by making cancer cells kill themselves, a process known among the scientific community as apoptosis.

The thing about polyphenols is that around 95% of them make it all the way to your colon without being digested. It is here that they're finally metabolized by microbiota in your gut, such as L. Bifidobacteria. Since polyphenols are a kind of nutrient for your microbiota, they promote the growth and abundance of the healthy ones in your gut. In fact, polyphenols are so good for your microbiome that medical professionals sometimes prescribe them as prebiotics. Polyphenols get along especially well with one type of bacteria called *Akkermansia muciniphila*. This microbiota is essential for preventing metabolic conditions like obesity and is particularly good at improving and strengthening your gut lining (Anhê et al., 2016).

Polyphenols are good for your healthy microbiota, not just Akkermansia muciniphila. To experience their full beneficial effects, you need to keep your diet as varied as possible. This way, you can consume as many different kinds of polyphenols as possible too. A great way to ensure this is to eat fruits and vegetables of all colors. As you may remember from our discussion of flavonoids, polyphenols are essentially fruit and vegetable pigments. This means that eating different colors of fruits and vegetables equals consuming different kinds of polyphenols, which is exactly what you should do.

Another micronutrient you want to make sure you consume plenty of is omega-3 fatty acids. Omega-3 fatty acids are a kind of polyunsaturated fat—the good fat you should eat more of—that, like polyphenols, has anti-inflammatory properties. On the whole, there are three types of omega-3s. These are (*Omega-3 Fatty Acids*, 2017)

- Alpha-linoleic acid (ALA)

- Docosahexaenoic acid (DHA)

- Eicosapentaenoic acid (EPA)

ALA is the most common omega-3 you'll likely consume because it's found in all sorts of things. Some examples are walnuts, flaxseed, soy, and canola. Interestingly enough, your body can convert DHA and EPA into ALA, albeit in small amounts. So again, ALA is the type of omega-3 you'll most often deal with. This is good news because ALA is vital for natural human growth and development, reduces your risk of developing heart disease of some sort, and prevents blood clots (*Alpha-Linolenic Acid (ALA)*, n.d.). However, this doesn't mean DHA and EPA are anything to scoff at. DHA is found in oily fishes, such as salmon and tuna. Studies indicate DHA can increase your focus, and it's known to be particularly helpful for people with ADHD (Juber, 2022). In pregnant women, it lowers the risk of experiencing a premature birth. In general, it improves your cardiovascular health, reduces inflammation throughout the body, and lowers your risk of developing an eye disease known as glaucoma.

As for EPA, it's mostly found in things like mussels and clams, though trout and herring also are rich in EPA. Like DHA, it lowers your risk of developing heart disease, lowers your triglyceride levels if they're high (also lowers high blood pressure), and prevents inflammation. It can even reduce the symptoms of depression, menopause, rheumatoid arthritis, and menstrual cramps (*Eicosapentaenoic Acid (EPA) Information*, n.d.).

So, how exactly do omega-3 fatty acids benefit your gut microbiome? First and foremost, omega-3s increase your gut microbiota's ability to produce short-chain fatty acids (Costantini et al., 2017). By now, you know enough about these to be aware of how important they are for your health. On top of that, omega-3s increase and promote microbiota diversity in your gut (Menni et al., 2017). As a result, it helps prevent conditions like colon cancer and IBD, as if all the benefits it was already offering weren't enough. Of course, omega-3s increase certain kinds of bacteria populations in your gut more than other types. The bacteria family they're most fond of is called Lachnospiraceae. This is a good thing because you want an abundance of bacteria from this family in your gut as they keep down inflammation and help lower your risk of developing a metabolic disease like obesity. Add to that how omega-3s make your gut less "leaky," and it's very easy to see why they should also be made a regular part of your diet.

Some foods you might not have thought should be a part of your diet but are absolutely vital for your gut health. Two examples of these might be mushrooms and bone broth. The thing about mushrooms is that they're very useful for increasing your gut microbiota diversity (Jayachandran et al., 2017). As before, you can choose from many kinds of yummy mushrooms, all of which have their own additional and unique benefits.

The most beneficial mushrooms you can go with for the sake of your gut health are

- **Shiitake**: These mushrooms have immense anti-inflammatory properties. They're great for protecting immune cells—especially those made in the gut—from any harmful pathogens that might have entered your system (Mishra et al., 2012).

- **Reishi**: Shiitake mushrooms aren't the only ones with anti-inflammatory properties. Reishi mushrooms can help you to keep inflammation levels down in your gut and across your body. In the process, it can prevent conditions like leaky gut, among other troubling conditions such as constipation and diarrhea, fatigue, and skin problems like eczema and psoriasis. Essentially, reiki mushrooms tighten your gut wall lining. An added bonus they bring to the table is that they can prevent ulcers from forming thanks to the presence of a bacteria called H. pylori.

- **Lion's mane**: Like reishi mushrooms, Lion's mane can also prevent the formation of ulcers. They are also good at keeping inflammation down and can prevent a wide array of intestinal disorders like ulcerative colitis. They can prevent other conditions aside from that, like cardiovascular diseases, for one. Lion's mane has even proven effective in combating certain mental health disorders such as depression and anxiety (Nagano et al., 2010).

- **Chaga:** These have been found to be particularly good deterrents against Crohn's disease. Actually, it's good for both types of IBD in terms of treating the condition and mitigating the crampy-painful symptoms that come with it. Positively brimming with antioxidants, Chaga mushrooms boost and strengthen your immunity while ensuring nothing is off with your digestion.

- **Turkey tail:** Adored by both the Bifidobacteria and Lactobacillus families, turkey tail is phenomenal for ensuring you have plenty of these little guys populating your guts (Eliza et al., 2012). They're equally as phenomenal in keeping the bad bacteria in your guts under control. Like various other mushrooms, they support your immune system, which is all thanks to the fact that they have a lot of fructooligosaccharides and prebiotic polysaccharides in them.

It's clear that mushrooms are unexpectedly good for your gut health, but how about bone broth? Bone broth is a nutritious soup stock made by simmering animal bones and connective tissues in plenty of water. It has been part of the human diet since time immemorial—

meaning it dates back to when our ancestors lived in caves. One of the great advantages of bone broth is that it's both easy to digest and makes digestion of all foods much easier. This is because bone broth has something called gelatin in it, which supports digestion. Gelatin is known to strengthen the mucosal lining of your gut walls, making it excellent for solving problems like having a leaky gut (Zhu et al., 2018).

A second component that can be found in bone broth is something called glutamine. Like gelatin, glutamine strengthens the mucosal lining of your gut wall, thereby helping to prevent chronic diseases that might occur as a result of having a leaky gut. Bone broth has a lot of amino acids in it too, which means that it comes with some strong anti-inflammatory properties (Razak et al., 2017). One of these amino acids is called arginine, and it is especially good at dealing with chronic inflammation.

Food to Avoid

Just as there are certain foods you should include in your diet to promote your gut health, there are certain foods you should try to avoid as much as possible. Removing these foods from your diet may be challenging, but you should strive to do so if you can. If you can't, then reducing your consumption as humanly possible will be a great start because they can be immensely damaging to your gut microbiome. The top food categories that you should make a point of avoiding are

- saturated fats

- soda

- red meat

- sugar

- alcohol

Saturated fats are an unhealthy kind of fat that's often found in things like meat products—think those white bits in bacon—and cheese. While you need to eat different kinds of fats, as a general rule, your diet shouldn't be too high in fats. This is because such a diet is sure to create an imbalance in your gut microbiome. A high-fat diet, you see, will reduce your firmicutes and Bacteroides populations. You need plenty of both in your gut because they help stave off inflammation and obesity.

Another reason you'll want to keep your saturated fat consumption to a minimum is because saturated fats change the bacterial makeup of your gut microbiome. This change typically results in your gut becoming inflamed, which in turn damages your intestinal tissues and can lead to health problems like IBD and colitis. In addition to that, saturated fats, which are found in things like baked goods and dairy products, promote the growth of a very harmful bacteria called *Bilophila wadsworthia* (Harmon, 2012). Bilophila is most often found in people who have IBD and other similar conditions and feeds off of sulfur, which is a byproduct of saturated fat consumption.

Soda is another food (or rather drink) to avoid for the sake of your gut health. As a rule, soft drinks are bad for your general health, especially those packed with sugar. They have absolutely no nutritional value, contribute significantly to weight gain, and increase liver fat by 27% (DiMeglio & Mattes, 2000). Like all that wasn't enough, they create dysbiosis in your gut microbiome in several ways. Soft drinks have artificial sweeteners in them. These sweeteners trigger your intestinal microbiota and lead to both metabolic issues and glucose intolerance in the process (Suez et al., 2014). They also interfere with your gut microbiota's day-to-day functions too (Bian et al., 2017).

Aside from all that, by now, numerous studies have linked soft drinks to type 2 diabetes, a metabolic disease that's related to the health and well-being of your gut microbiota. It has also been linked to insulin resistance (Mathur et al., 2020). These findings make it easy to see why avoiding soft drinks is a good idea.

As for red meat, while you don't have to quit it altogether, reducing how often you eat it is a good idea. So far, many studies have uncovered connections between red meat and colon cancer and heart diseases, among other health problems. Scientists aren't entirely sure why this is the case, but the most likely culprit is N-glycolylneuraminic acid (Neu5G). Neu5G, which sounds like a new iPhone model, is a kind of sugar molecule that human beings cannot naturally produce (Bryant, 2019). It is, however, a molecule that can be incorporated into their cells when they eat red meat, which does contain it in droves. The problem with this is that the human body considers Neu5G as a foreign substance and therefore attacks it. This causes inflammation in the gut, which inevitably leads to health issues like colon cancer.

Of course, this wouldn't happen if you didn't have bacteria that release the enzymes necessary to extract Neu5G from red meat and work it into your cells. Sadly, you do have such bacteria among the hundreds that populate your guts. This situation can be mitigated if scientists ever find a way to prevent that enzyme—known as sialic acid—from tangling with Neu5G. Unfortunately, they are nowhere near achieving this, so it's a good idea to keep your red meat consumption low for the time being.

Of all the food items out there, the thing you most want to avoid to maintain your gut and overall health is sugar. Sugar is very damaging to you in too many ways to count. It must be noted, though, that there are two types of sugar: Fructose and sucrose. Fructose is the kind of sugar you naturally find in things like fruits, and it's actually good for you. Studies have found that fructose supports the health and growth of beneficial bacteria in your gut, like B. thetaiotaomicron. Sucrose, on the other hand, does the opposite. Far from being beneficial for your healthy gut microbiota, sucrose (or table sugar as it's commonly known) blocks the production of protein in your body (Hathaway, 2018). In doing so, it contributes to weight gain problems and metabolic issues. While it's at it, sucrose gets to work, eliminating the good bacteria from your gut. This makes your gut microbiome imbalanced, which, interestingly enough, makes you crave even more sugar. The more you crave, the more sugar you eat, and before you know it, you're enjoying sugary snacks every day, continually harming your gut microbiome in the process.

Sucrose, being what it is, is well known for being directly connected to your risk of developing diabetes. However, did you know that it also plays a part in leaky gut syndrome? It turns out that because eating too much sugar kills off the good bacteria in your gut, your intestinal mucosal barrier starts weakening. Thus, more unwanted toxic materials leak into your bloodstream, leading to even more health problems in the long run.

Cutting sucrose from your diet is one of the best things you can do for yourself and your gut microbiome. The same might be said about alcohol, which is again known to create dysbiosis in the gut if you consume it regularly.

Chapter 7:

Gut Microbiota and the
Future of Health

As you've no doubt noticed throughout this book, plenty of scientists are conducting a lot of research about the gut microbiome. This is to be expected. After all, the gut microbiome is a vast and complicated environment. One thing that scientists have discovered in their research is that gut microbiota can be used in several ways to treat different conditions. This realization has led to the creation of probiotic and prebiotic supplements. These supplements, though, aren't the only ways in which the gut microbiota can be utilized to fix health problems and improve your health. From fecal transplants to psychobiotics, the gut microbiota can be used in some staggering ways. These are only the beginning of what might be achieved using such microbiota, as you'll soon discover for yourself.

Fecal Transplants

I can almost hear you asking yourself, "What on earth is a fecal transplant?" And see you scrunch up your face at the likely image the term conjures up. Said images aren't as accurate as you think, though. Like you probably suspect, fecal transplants have to do with feces. The idea here is to collect fecal samples—yes, meaning poop—from someone with a healthy and balanced gut microbiome. You can then introduce the sample you've collected to a patient's GI tract. This procedure is usually done for one of two reasons: To restore the patient's healthy gut microbiome and to treat a condition known as Clostridium difficile, otherwise known as C. diff (Fecal Transplant, 2022).

C. diff is a condition that can occur after you've taken a round of antibiotics. As useful as they can be, antibiotics, unfortunately, kill off a lot of good bacteria in your gut. As a result, the bad bacteria there flourish, and one of these bacteria is known as C. diff, which is a rather unpleasant microorganism that can cause symptoms such as bad cramping, diarrhea, and a high fever.

Regardless of which of the two conditions you're undergoing a fecal transplant for, the procedure will be done during a colonoscopy. During said colonoscopy, a gastroenterologist will guide a colonoscope through your colon. As the colonoscope is withdrawn, the sample that it was carrying will be left inside the colon. This is the most common way of performing a fecal transplant, but it's not the only one. Another (albeit much less common) way is to insert a tube down the nose of the patient and have it go all the way down to the point where their stomach connects to their small intestines. It is here that the sample will be deposited. However, this method is generally not preferred because it comes with a rather high risk of aspiration pneumonia.

How do you know the donor has a healthy microbiome, though? You check that they meet certain standards, of course. For example, if someone is donating a fecal sample, they must not have been on any antibiotic prescriptions for at least six months. They must not be at risk for an infectious disease or be immunocompromised either. Likewise, they cannot be someone who is living with gastrointestinal conditions like IBD since those will be major indicators of an unhealthy microbiome anyway. If the donor meets those criteria, they will further be screened for other conditions such as HIV, C. diff, and syphilis. If they pass this screening, it will be time for the preparation stage.

The preparation stage is fairly simple for the done, in all honesty. First, they will be asked if they're on any medication and if they have any allergies. Second, they will need to go off any antibiotic medication they may be on for at least two days before they receive their transplant. Similarly, they may need to stop other medication that they're on, depending on what their doctor suggests. If the donee will be receiving their sample via colonoscopy, they will be given a bowel prep regime to follow. This may entail a couple of different things, like an enema (fun!) or an all-liquid diet for a few days. If they'll be receiving their sample via endoscopy—meaning through the tube in their nose—they'll need to be put under, and understandably so.

As for what happens during the actual procedure itself, that depends on which method is being used. For the colonoscopy method, the gastroenterologist will mix the sample in question with a saline solution until everything is in a liquid state. When the mixture is ready, you'll be given a sedative (though you won't be put under), and the doctor will guide the sample where it needs to go; your colon. After the procedure is complete, you will be allowed to return home. You may also receive a prescription for an antidiuretic to enhance the effectiveness of the transplant. If you've gone with the through-the-nose method, then you'll be given anesthesia and likely will have to stay in the hospital for a short while and then be taken home by someone you trust.

While fecal transplants are safe, they can have some side effects, just as any medical procedure can. These side effects are generally on the mild side, though, and include:

- Bloating and gassiness.

- Constipation, thanks to the antidiuretic you're taking.

- The transplant solution leaking out just a tiny bit.

- Cramping if any air got trapped in your intestines during the procedure.

Some of the more serious side effects that may occur are:

- Pneumonia if the sample was delivered through the nose.

- Infection if the transplant sample was compromised or wasn't adequately tested.

- Infection from any tearing or bleeding that may have happened during the procedure.

If you experience any of these latter complications, you should see your doctor about them immediately.

Psychobiotics For Treating Depression

You already know that there's a firmly established link between your gut microbiota and mental health disorders like depression. That being the case, it shouldn't be too surprising to hear that scientists have begun exploring a new treatment method for depression that utilizes the power of gut microbiota, known as psychobiotics. Psychobiotics are a kind of probiotics that affect the central nervous system. As a result, they impact things like your mood and behavior by using the gut-brain axis. The idea here is that by taking the right psychobiotics and thus fixing things like your gut permeability, hormone signals, and gut immune system, you'll be able to influence your brain chemistry. In doing so, you'll be able to impact the severity and symptoms of your depressive disorder.

If you're skeptical about whether or not psychobiotics work, initial evidence indicates that they do (Dinan et al., 2013). Psychobiotics are apparently effective against both depression and chronic fatigue syndrome, and this is more than likely related to the anti-inflammatory properties that accompany them. It may also have to do with how psychobiotics reduce the activity levels seen in your hypothalamic-pituitary-adrenal axis, which play an important part in encouraging anxiety and depressive symptoms.

In addition to all this, further studies indicate that psychobiotics can be effectively used to treat stress—especially chronic stress. When you feel stressed, your body becomes flooded with the stress hormone known as cortisol. Cortisol blocks your immune system and makes your guts more permeable, leading to the infamous leaky gut syndrome. Taking psychobiotics, however, reverses all this and brings your stress levels down, thereby cutting off the flood of cortisol in your body. Fixing the leakiness of your gut walls isn't just important for the sake of your stress levels but for your depression as well. Additionally, studies show that depression is also linked with gut permeability (Trzeciak & Herbet, 2021). As a general rule, the less "leaky" your guts are, the more physically and mentally healthy you'll be.

Gut Bacteria Can Improve Your Memory

Seeing as your gut microbiota can prevent degenerative conditions, particularly those related to aging, it stands to reason that you can use them to improve various cognitive functions like your memory. While the research exploring the gut microbiome-memory connection is still in its infancy, its findings seem to be quite promising. One study, for example, has found that ingesting the kinds of bacteria found in certain probiotics can greatly improve long-term memory (O'Hagan et al., 2017). Granted, the said study was done with mice and their ability to recall how to properly navigate mazes. Still, as initial results go, it's quite promising.

Most of the studies conducted on this matter indicate that the most useful bacteria for improving memory is the Lactobacillus genus. It's not for nothing that it's been discovered that this same bacteria genus improves memory and cognition among Alzheimer's patients (Akbari et al., 2201).

Gut Microbiota Can Rebuild Your Immune System

One interesting thing you can use your gut microbiota for is improving and even rebuilding your immune system (Sanfins, 2020). The fact that there's a firm connection between your gut microbiota and your immune system is undeniable at this point. Logically speaking, that connection is something that you can (and should) leverage for your health. This is especially true if you've undergone treatments such as chemotherapy that are known to destroy immune systems alongside the cancers they're trying to kill off.

Normally, you would need a bone marrow treatment after you're done with things like chemotherapy or radiotherapy and are officially cancer-free. A bone marrow transplant is where you're injected with healthy stem cells taken from a healthy individual's bone marrow. If you recall, those cells then replenish your ability to make white blood cells, which are the powerhouses of your immune system. While these cells will help you to rebuild your immune system, you'll still be vulnerable to various infections the first few weeks after your bone marrow transplant. Given that, you'll have to take antibiotics as a safety measure. The problem is that those antibiotics will kill off the healthy bacteria in your gut while giving you the protection you lack and need (Schluter et al., 2020). So, they constitute a bit of a good news-bad news scenario.

In this situation, your gut microbiota can come into the picture in the form of certain probiotics after you're done with your round of antibiotics. Of these microbiota, taking supplements or pills to be taken in the form of three specific ones—Akkermansia, Faecalibacterium, and Ruminococcus-2—will be especially helpful to you. Scientists have found that these three microbiota are most closely associated with increased numbers of immune cells in the blood when it comes to patients recovering from chemo and antibiotic treatments.

Predicting The Development Of Neurological and Metabolic Diseases

Aside from being used as various methods of treatment, your gut microbiota can be used as disease markers, so to speak. Imagine that you went to the doctor for a regular checkup, and your doctor asked you for a fecal sample. You provided such a sample, and it was screened. You and your doctor are now sitting in his office, going over the results. The results show exactly which microbiota were present in your stool and their levels. Depending on those levels, your doctor identifies certain "bad" bacteria in your stool. Maybe these bacteria are indicative of your risk of developing diabetes. Maybe they point to your being in the risk group for acquiring a cardiovascular disease of some sort. Maybe they point toward a neurological or metabolic disease.

Whatever the findings are, once your doctor spots these markers, they can make the right recommendations for you to avert or mitigate the disease in question. This might mean prescribing certain specific probiotics or prebiotics to you. It might mean encouraging you to eat more of certain kinds of foods or to change your diet entirely. Whatever the case, the reality at hand is simple: The kinds and quantities of microbiota in your gut can be used as disease markers. As such, they can help you prevent certain diseases and serve as treatments if you are already struggling with them.

Of course, for this scenario to become a reality, scientists must first identify all the different microbiota in our guts and exactly what they do in their various quantities. While they have made significant headway in this regard, let's be honest, we are still at the very beginning of their endeavors. Hence, figuring out how to use microbiota as disease biomarkers and using that information will take a while. In the meantime, you're just going to have to watch what you eat, which you now can do since you know what foods are good for you, and support your gut microbiome by taking certain supplements. Speaking of what to eat, what do you need to eat to maintain your gut health? Let's find out by taking a look at some sample meals.

Chapter 8:

Eat Your Way to a Healthy Gut

You might be a little unsure how to go about planning gut-healthy meals. If so, fear not. Here's a sample, easy-to-prepare meal plan that you can turn to in a crunch!

The Seven-Day Meal Plan

Monday

Breakfast: Kefir-Berry Smoothie

Prep Time: 5 minutes

Total Time: 5 minutes

Nutritional Facts/Info:

- *Calories: 304 cal.*
- *Fats: 7 grams*

- *Carbs: 53 grams*

- *Protein: 15 grams*

Ingredients:

- 1 cup of kefir

- 1 ½ cups of berries of your choice

- ½ a banana

- 2 teaspoons of cashew or peanut butter

Instructions:

1. Take out your food processor.

2. Place all the ingredients into the processor and turn it on. Keep blending until the texture becomes as smooth as you'd like.

3. Pour into a glass or bowl and enjoy.

Lunch: Kale Salad with Chicken and Quinoa

Prep Time: 10 minutes

Total Time: 10 minutes

Nutrition Facts/Info:

- *Calories: 301 cal.*

- *Fats: 8 grams*

- *Carbs: 30 grams*
- *Protein: 27 grams*

Ingredients:

- 1 bag of chopped kale
- 1 ½ cups of cooked quinoa
- 1 cup of shredded and grilled chicken
- 1 chopped cucumber
- ¼ cup pitted black olives
- 1 chopped medium tomato
- ¼ cup of crumbled feta cheese
- ¼ cup of Greek salad dressing

Instructions:

1. Mix the kale, quinoa, black olives, cucumbers, and tomatoes in a medium-sized bowl.
2. Drizzle the Greek salad dressing over it and mix well.
3. Sprinkle the crumbled feta cheese over the bowl, then serve and enjoy with salt to taste.

Dinner: Honey Garlic Salmon

Prep Time: 10 minutes

Cook Time: 15-20 minutes

Total Time: 25-40 minutes

Nutrition Facts/Info:

- *Calories: 222 cal.*
- *Fats: 9 grams*
- *Carbs: 5 grams*
- *Protein: 29 grams*

Ingredients

- 1 medium-sized salmon
- 2 tablespoons of low-sodium soy sauce
- 2 cloves of minced garlic
- 1 tablespoon of honey

Instructions:

1. Mix the low-sodium soy sauce, minced garlic, and honey in a bowl.
2. Pour the mixture into sealable plastic bags, leaving enough room for the salmon to fit into them without the mixture spilling out. This

should equal about three to four tablespoons of sauce.

3. Place the individual salmon into the sealable plastic bags and place the bags into the fridge so that the fish can marinate in the sauce.

4. Turn the bags once every five minutes to ensure that the salmons are thoroughly soaked in the sauce. Let the fish marinate for 20 minutes.

5. Preheat the oven to broil.

6. Take the salmon from the fridge, out of the bags they're in, and place them on a baking tray lined with a baking sheet.

7. Pour the remaining sauce in the bags over the fish before sprinkling some salt over them.

8. Place the fish in the oven and let them broil for 15-20 minutes.

Tuesday

Breakfast: Avocado and Strawberry Toast

Prep Time: 5 minutes

Cook Time: 5 minutes

Total Time: 10 minutes

Nutrition Facts/Info:

- *Calories: 177 cal.*
- *Fats: 9 grams*
- *Carbs: 35 grams*
- *Protein: 12 grams*

Ingredients:

- 2 slices of toasted whole-grain bread
- ½ smashed avocado
- Sliced strawberries (as many as you would like)

Instructions:

1. Toast your whole-grain bread.
2. Peel and pit your avocado and slice it in half.
3. Mash the avocado until it takes on a spreadable quality.
4. Spread the avocado mash over the toasted bread.
5. Top the avocado with the sliced strawberries, and enjoy.

Lunch: Veggie and Hummus Pita Pockets

Prep Time: 5 minutes

Cook Time: 30 minutes

Total Time: 35 minutes

Nutrition Facts/Info:

- *Calories: 357 cal.*
- *Fats: 12 grams*
- *Carbs: 54 grams*
- *Protein: 14 grams*

Ingredients:

- 1 whole wheat pita bread
- 4-5 tbsp. of hummus
- ½ cup of diced oven-roasted carrots, shallots, and onions
- ½ cup of salad greens
- ¼ cup of roasted peppers

Instructions:

1. Slice your pita bread in half.
2. Preheat the oven to 425°F.

3. Dice your carrots, shallots, peppers, and onions and toss in a medium-sized bowl.

4. Drizzle 2 tbsp. of olive oil over them and add a pinch of salt, along with the herbs of your choice. Mix well until all the vegetables are coated in it.

5. Bake the vegetables for about 30 minutes.

6. Spread 2 tbsp. of hummus on each half of the sliced pita bread.

7. Take out the roasted vegetables from the oven and divide them evenly between the pita breads.

8. Serve while hot or warm, and enjoy.

Dinner: Spinach and Tomato Orzo Salad

Prep Time: 15 minutes

Cook Time: 15-20 minutes

Total Time: 30-35 minutes

Nutrition Facts/Info:

- *Calories: 129 cal.*
- *Fats: 1 gram*
- *Carbs: 26 grams*
- *Protein: 5 grams*

Ingredients:

- 1 ½ cups of cooked orzo
- 8 oz. of cherry tomatoes
- 2 minced garlic cloves
- 4 cups of fresh baby spinach
- 2 chopped green onions
- 1 lemon, juiced
- 1 tsp. of dried basil
- 2 tbsp of olive oil
- a pinch of salt to taste
- ¼ cup of feta cheese crumbles or diced mozzarella.

Instructions:

1. In a pot, bring ¼ cup of water to a boil.
2. Once the water is boiling, pour in the orzo and cook for about 8 minutes.
3. Pour in the fresh baby spinach and cook for an additional 1-2 minutes.
4. Drain the mixture and gently rinse the orzo and spinach in cool water. Then place them in a medium-sized bowl.

5. Add in the cherry tomatoes and green onions. Stir.

6. Add in the garlic, lemon juice, basil, olive oil, and salt. Keep stirring until everything is well-mixed.

7. Top with the cheese of your choice and serve.

Wednesday

Breakfast: Pecan-Blueberry Overnight Oatmeal

Prep Time: 8 hours (overnight)

Cook Time: 10 minutes

Total Time: 8 hours + 10 minutes

Nutrition Facts/Info:

- *Calories: 291 cal.*
- *Fats: 8 grams*
- *Carbs: 49 grams*
- *Protein: 9 grams*

Ingredients:

- ½ cup of rolled oats
- ½ cup of water

- ½ cup of blueberries (or berries of your choice)
- 2-3 tbsp. of nonfat Greek yogurt
- 1-2 tbsp. of pecans
- 2 tbsp. of maple syrup or honey

Instructions:

1. In a cup, small bowl, or mason jar, mix the oats, water, and salt.
2. Cover the mixture with something like a lid and leave it in the fridge overnight.
3. Take out the mixture in the morning and top it with pecans, blueberries, yogurt, and maple syrup or honey.
4. Serve and enjoy.

Lunch: Kimchi Shrimp Noodles

Prep Time: 10 minutes

Cook Time: 20-30 minutes

Total Time: 30-40 minutes

Nutrition Facts/Info:

- *Calories: 570 cal.*
- *Fats: 17 grams*

- *Carbs: 73 grams*

- *Protein: 32 grams*

Ingredients:

- 1 ½ cup of chopped cabbage
- 2 minced garlic cloves
- 1 oz. of fresh, chopped ginger
- 1 ½ cups of cooked noodles
- 2 sprigs of spring onions
- 2 tbsp. of fish sauce
- 2 tbsp. of cilantro
- 3 slices of lime
- 20 oz. of shrimp
- 1 packet of chickpea pasta
- 2 oz. of gochujang

Instructions:

1. Take 3 canning jars and divide the gochujang evenly between them.
2. Cook the noodles.
3. Add ½ a cup of cabbage, ¼ cup of kimchi, 3 oz. of shrimp, and ½ cup of noodles into each jar, layering them in the given order.

4. Top each jar with cilantro, divided evenly between them, along with one lime per jar.

5. Cover the jars with their lids and place them in the fridge. Let them sit there for up to three days.

6. When you remove a jar from the fridge, pour one cup of very hot water into it, cover it again, and shake well.

7. Remove the lid and place the jar in the microwave. Cook for 1 minute on high. Do this twice more if it's not steaming hot.

8. Set the jar on the counter and let it cool for about 3 minutes.

9. Serve and enjoy.

Dinner: Squash Spaghetti with Avocado Pesto Sauce

Prep Time: 10 minutes

Cook Time: 5-7 minutes

Total Time: 15-17 minutes

Nutrition Facts/Info:

- *Calories: 362 cal.*

- *Fats: 34.1 grams*
- *Carbs: 16 grams*
- *Protein: 4.6 grams*

Ingredients:

- 1 ripe avocado, peeled and diced
- ½ cup of fresh basil leaves
- ¼ cup of shelled pistachios
- 2 cloves of minced garlic
- 1 tbsp. of lime juice
- 1 oz. of squash pasta
- 3 tbsp. of olive oil
- Enough water to cover the pasta
- Salt and pepper to taste

Instructions:

1. Preheat the oven to 400°F.
2. Thinly slice the squash and spread them across a baking tray lined with a baking sheet.
3. Bake the squash for about 45 minutes.
4. Place the garlic, avocado, lime juice, pistachios, salt, and pepper in a food processor.

5. Turn the food processor on until everything becomes finely chopped. Add in the olive oil and turn the processor on again until the mixture is smooth.

6. Remove the squash from the oven and place in a bowl. Top with the pesto sauce you made, and enjoy.

Thursday

Breakfast: Kefir-Berry Smoothie

Nutrition Facts/Info:

- *Calories: 304 cal.*
- *Fats: 7 grams*
- *Carbs: 53 grams*
- *Protein: 15 grams*

Ingredients:

- 1 cup of kefir
- 1 ½ cups of the berry of your choice
- ½ a banana
- 2 teaspoons of cashew or peanut butter

Lunch: Stuffed Sweet Potato

Prep Time: 10 minutes

Cook Time: 45-50 minutes

Total Time: 55 minutes-1 hour

Nutrition Facts/Info:

- *Calories: 401 cal.*
- *Fats: 9 grams*
- *Carbs: 66 grams*
- *Protein: 12 grams*

Ingredients:

- 5 sweet potatoes
- ⅓ cup of cooked quinoa
- 1 diced onion
- 1 diced chive
- 1 finely diced and seeded jalapeno pepper
- 3 cloves of minced garlic
- 1 tsp. of chili powder (more if you'd like it spicier)
- ½ tsp. of ground cumin
- 1 can of black beans, rinsed
- 1 cup of shredded cheddar cheese

- 2 tbsp. of lemon juice
- salsa and guacamole to serve

Instructions:

1. Stab your sweet potatoes repeatedly with a fork. Microwave them on high for about 10 minutes.

2. Cook the quinoa.

3. Rinse the beans and cook them in a pot over medium-high heat while continually stirring.

4. Dice the onions, chives, and peppers, and then roast them in a pan with olive oil and garlic until they become tender.

5. Mix the cooked beans with the roasted vegetables.

6. Split the potatoes in half and divide the mixture evenly between them, pouring it into the space you formed.

7. Top with salsa and guac, and enjoy.

Dinner: Spinach and Tomato Orzo Salad

Nutrition Facts/Info:

- *Calories: 129 cal.*
- *Fats: 1 gram*

- *Carbs: 26 grams*
- *Protein: 5 grams*

Ingredients:

- 1 ½ cups of cooked orzo
- 8 oz. of cherry tomatoes
- 2 minced garlic cloves
- 4 cups of fresh baby spinach
- 2 chopped green onions
- 1 lemon, juiced
- 1 tsp. of dried basil
- 2 tbsp of olive oil
- a pinch of salt to taste
- ¼ cup of feta cheese crumbles or diced mozzarella.

Friday

Breakfast: Avocado Toast with Strawberries

Nutrition Facts/Info:

- *Calories: 177 cal.*
- *Fats: 9 grams*

- *Carbs: 35 grams*
- *Protein: 12 grams*

Ingredients:

- 2 slices of toasted whole-grain bread
- ½ a smashed avocado
- Sliced strawberries (as many as you would like)

Lunch: Kale Salad with Chicken and Quinoa

Nutrition Facts/Info:

- *Calories: 301 cal.*
- *Fats: 8 grams*
- *Carbs: 30 grams*
- *Protein: 27 grams*

Ingredients:

- 1 bag of chopped kale
- 1 ½ cups of cooked quinoa
- 1 cup of shredded and grilled chicken
- 1 chopped cucumber
- ¼ cup pitted black olives
- 1 chopped, medium tomato
- ¼ cup of feta cheese crumbles

- ¼ cup of Greek salad dressing

Dinner: Honey Garlic Salmon

Prep Time: 10 minutes

Cook Time: 15-20 minutes

Total Time: 25-40 minutes

Nutrition Facts/Info:

- *Calories: 222 cal.*
- *Fats: 9 grams*
- *Carbs: 5 grams*
- *Protein: 29 grams*

Ingredients

- 1 medium-sized salmon
- 2 tablespoons of low-sodium soy sauce
- 2 cloves of minced garlic
- 1 tablespoon of honey

Saturday

Breakfast: Banana and Peanut Butter Toast

Prep Time: 5 minutes

Total Time: 5 minutes

Nutrition Facts/Info:

- *Calories: 346 cal.*
- *Fats: 20.3 grams*
- *Carbs: 46.8 grams*
- *Protein: 16.3 grams*

Ingredients:

- 2 slices of toasted whole-grain bread
- 1 diced banana
- 2 tbsp. of peanut butter
- 1 tsp. of honey to glaze over

Instructions:

1. Toast your bread.
2. Spread 1 tbsp. Of peanut butter over each slice.
3. Dice your banana.
4. Place the diced bits over the slices that are covered with peanut butter.

5. Drizzle some honey over them and enjoy.

Lunch: Kimchi Shrimp Noodles

Nutrition Facts/Info:

- *Calories: 570 cal.*
- *Fats: 17 grams*
- *Carbs: 73 grams*
- *Protein: 32 grams*

Ingredients:

- 1 ½ cup of chopped cabbage
- 2 minced garlic cloves
- 1 oz. of fresh, chopped ginger
- 1 ½ cups of cooked noodles
- 2 sprigs of spring onions
- 2 tbsp. of fish sauce
- 2 tbsp. of cilantro
- 3 slices of lime
- 20 oz. of shrimp
- 1 packet of chickpea pasta
- 2 oz. of gochujang

Dinner: Squash Spaghetti with Avocado Pesto Sauce

Nutrition Facts/Info:

- *Calories: 362 cal.*
- *Fats: 34.1 grams*
- *Carbs: 16 grams*
- *Protein: 4.6 grams*

Ingredients:

- 1 ripe avocado, peeled and diced
- ½ cup of fresh basil leaves
- ¼ cup of shelled pistachios
- 2 cloves of minced garlic
- 1 tbsp. of lime juice
- 1 oz. of squash pasta
- 3 tbsp. of olive oil
- Enough water to cover the pasta
- Salt and pepper to taste

Sunday

Breakfast: Pecan-Blueberry Overnight Oatmeal

Nutrition Facts/Info:

- *Calories: 291 cal.*
- *Fats: 8 grams*
- *Carbs: 49 grams*
- *Protein: 9 grams*

Ingredients:

- ½ cup of rolled oats
- ½ cup of water
- ½ cup of blueberries (or berries of your choice)
- 2-3 tbsp. of nonfat Greek yogurt
- 1-2 tbsp. of pecans
- 2 tbsp. of maple syrup or honey

Lunch: Veggie and Hummus Pita Pockets

Nutrition Facts/Info:

- *Calories: 357 cal.*
- *Fats: 12 grams*
- *Carbs: 54 grams*

- *Protein: 14 grams*

Ingredients:

- 1 whole wheat pita bread
- 4-5 tbsp. of hummus
- ½ cup of diced oven-roasted and diced carrots, shallots, and onions
- ½ cup of salad greens
- ¼ cup of roasted peppers

Dinner: Lemon Linguine

Prep Time: 10 minutes

Cook Time: 20 minutes

Total Time: 30 minutes

Nutrition Facts/Info:

- *Calories: 372 cal.*
- *Fats: 7 grams*
- *Carbs: 64 grams*
- *Protein: 18 grams*

Ingredients:

- 1 packet of whole wheat linguine

- 3 cloves of minced garlic

- 3 ½ cups of water

- 1 packet of artichoke hearts

- 6 cups of spinach

- 3 tbsp. of lemon juice

- ½ cup of grated parmesan cheese

Instructions:

1. Pour the water into a pot and bring it to a boil.

2. Add in the pasta, garlic, and oil, and keep boiling for 8 minutes.

3. Stir in the spinach and artichokes. Keep boiling for 4 minutes more.

4. Remove from heat and drain.

5. Add in the lemon juice and parmesan. Stir and let it sit for 5 minutes.

6. Serve and enjoy with salt and pepper to taste.

Pick and Mix

One of the key things to remember when you're crafting your meal plan is that you need to incorporate as many different healthy ingredients into it as you can. As a rule of thumb, your gut microbiome loves food diversity. It needs it in order to be diverse. Keep this fact in mind as you're planning out your meals. Try to eat different kinds of dishes for lunch and dinner and on alternating days. This will both be good for your gut microbiome and, let's face it, keep you from getting bored.

Another thing you might want to keep in mind for your gut health is the importance of mindful eating. We often eat our food way too quickly, especially if we're watching a show as we eat or something like that. The problem with this is that it prevents the enzymes in your saliva from doing their job, which is to help with digestion (Boyers, 2022). Not chewing your food thoroughly can make things harder on your gut and your gut microbiome, resulting in inflammation, bloating, gas, and other similar symptoms that you want to avoid.

Dietary Adjustments For Digestive Issues

While the varied diet that we've discussed (and even given some examples of) is good for general gut health, it might not be the best fit for people with certain digestive disorders like IBD, sucrose intolerance, and Small Intestine Bacterial Overgrowth. If you have one of these disorders, it's important that you know exactly how you should eat to maintain your gut microbiome health.

If you've IBD, then that means you're experiencing symptoms such as diarrhea. With such symptoms, it's important that you keep the fluid levels in your gut low.

This is because more fluid in your guts means changes in the speed at which your food will be ingested and metabolized by your gut microbiota (*Try a FODMAPs Diet to Manage Irritable Bowel Syndrome*, 2014). High fluid levels in your gut will result in more gas and bloatedness, among other things. In an effort to avoid such a thing, you need to eat fewer foods containing Lactose, Fructose, Fructans, GOS, and polyols.

What does that leave, then? Plenty! If we're talking fruits, eating bananas, kiwi, oranges, strawberries, and grapefruit, as well as other citruses, will be very helpful for IBD. If we're talking vegetables, you should go for carrots, bean sprouts, potatoes, parsnips, olives, and chives, to name a few examples. You can also eat certain dairy products as long as they're lactose-free. Lactose-free milk is always an option, as are hard cheeses like feta. At the top of the list of proteins that are beneficial to your gut health are eggs, tofu, beef, chicken, and fish. Nuts should be limited to 10 to 15 pieces a day when you have IBD, though no such rule applies to grains. You can go with things like oat bran, gluten-free pasta and rice, and quinoa.

Of these, oats will prove a particularly helpful remedy against bloating (*Diet, Lifestyle and Medicines - Irritable Bowel Syndrome (IBD)*, 2019). The same can be said for linseeds, which you can eat about a spoonful of per day. Meanwhile, cutting back on high-fiber foods like whole grains should help with diarrhea. In contrast, if you're struggling with constipation, the doctor's orders are to drink lots of water and eat more fiber-rich foods like potatoes and carrots.

Sucrose intolerance is a condition that happens because your gut and your gut microbiome have become damaged, leading to digestive disorders. As a result of this damage, your gut microbiome isn't able to produce the enzyme needed to digest sucrose, which is known as sucrase (Burkhart, 2020). It's that undigested sucrose that gets left over in your guts that causes the troubling symptoms that come with the disorder. These symptoms are experiencing diarrhea after eating, bloating, abdominal cramps, and smelly gas.

The ideal diet for sucrose intolerance comprises food that doesn't contain sucrose. Finding such food is relatively easy, as long as you remember to check the labels of the foods you're purchasing. After all, you don't want any added sugar in the yogurt you buy—or anything else like that. A low-sucrose diet also means being mindful about which fruits you consume, as some have higher sucrose contents than others. For example, cherries, strawberries, and kiwi are very low in sucrose but very tasty regardless. On the other hand, pineapples, apples, and cantaloupes are high in sucrose and, thus, should be avoided.

Lastly, there's Small Intestine Bacterial Overgrowth (SIBO). As per the name, SIBO is a condition where various bacteria overgrow in your small intestine, in stark contrast to the rest of your digestive tract (Anthony, 2018). The condition can be rather painful as it can cause malnutrition and diarrhea, and if left untreated, it can result in you having to have surgery and cause nerve damage in your small intestine.

The first thing your doctor will do when you're given a SIBO diagnosis is to put you on a round of antibiotics, given their ability to kill off the bacteria in your gut. The second thing they'll do is switch you to a specific diet made up of foods devoid of the nutrients that those overgrown bacteria like to feast on and ferment. The nutrients to avoid in this regard are sucrose, fiber, sugar alcohol, and inulin. Interestingly enough, the diet you'd adopt to take care of a sucrose intolerance would also work very well for tending to SIBO. In keeping with that, some examples of foods you'd want to eat more of are:

- Fish

- Eggs

- Meat

- Broccoli

- Carrots

- Leafy greens

- Oatmeal

- Squash

- Potatoes

- Grapes

- Strawberries

- Olives

- Peanuts

- Pumpkin

Additionally, the foods you want to avoid are

- Apples
- Dried fruit of any type
- High fructose corn syrup
- Honey and agave
- Soft drinks
- Butternut squash
- Artichokes
- Asparagus
- Onions
- Garlic
- Beans
- Cauliflower
- Ice cream
- Sweetened cereals
- Baked goods
- Flavored or sweetened yogurt
- Rye, barley, and grains
- Peas

As long as you keep these rules in mind, you should be able to regain your gut health thanks to the food you eat and take the first necessary step to adopt the kind of lifestyle that's good for your gut microbiome.

Chapter 9:

Live a Gut-Healthy
Lifestyle

Leading a healthy, happy, and long life starts with eating a healthy diet. That much is known. However, it's also known that a healthy diet goes hand in hand with regular exercise. When combined, these two things contribute immeasurably to your well-being. Regular exercise is something that can be considered a part of your lifestyle choices, and your lifestyle choices are the second key to improving your gut health. Things like your day-to-day activity level, your sleep schedule, and stress management techniques impact your gut microbiome pretty directly, whether you realize it or not. Making lifestyle changes is something you can do regardless of what age you are. Moreover, at times it can be something you absolutely have to do to live the kind of healthy life you deserve.

Fix Your Sleep Schedule

Like with your brain, your gut microbiome has a bidirectional relationship with your sleep schedule, meaning that the two affect one another. Poor sleeping habits can negatively impact your gut microbiome and result in digestive issues. Said digestive issues can then make it difficult for you to either fall asleep or they can continually wake you up throughout the night, thus interfering with the quality of your sleep (Farah, 2022).

Truthfully, your gut microbiome affects your sleep cycle in a couple of different ways. As you learned, some of the microbiota in your gut produce something called butyrate. You need to have sufficient rates of butyrate in your system because, as it turns out, this chemical enhances the quality of your sleep (Sen et al., 2021). According to one study, when you have higher rates of butyrate in your system, the quality of your sleep at certain stages (like deep sleep, for example) improves and increases by as much as 50-70% (Szentirmai et al., 2019).

Another way in which your gut microbiota impact your sleep has to do with your circadian rhythms. You see, the bacteria from the Lactobacillus genus in your gut can directly influence your circadian rhythms. When there's dysbiosis in your gut microbiome and your Lactobacillus quantities go down as a result, your circadian rhythms become irregular (Bishehsari et al., 2020). This is because the existing imbalance messes with both your internal clock and the genes regulating your circadian rhythms.

All this has nothing on the stress that lack of sleep can cause throughout your body. As a general rule, chronic stress is not good for your health and is especially bad for your gut microbiome. This, of course, has to do with the fact your cortisol levels rise when you're stressed and adversely affect your gut microbiome, sometimes even causing you to develop leaky gut syndrome.

You can do several things to improve the quality and duration of your sleep. One is to avoid big meals before you go to bed. As a general rule, you should have stopped eating approximately three hours before bedtime. This goes doubly for drinking coffee or any other caffeinated drinks late at night. That way, you won't burden your digestive system when it's supposed to be resting— after all, every living being and organism needs rest—and those digestive processes won't interrupt your sleep.

Stay Stress-Free

Stress can be caused by many different things. While momentary stress is a part of everyday life and is fairly normal, it becomes a huge issue when it gets to be chronic. As mentioned before, this has to do with the amount of cortisol, the stress hormone, released in your body at such times. When you get stressed, your sympathetic nervous system kicks into gear and sends a message down to your gut, telling it to stop operations. The idea here is to stop all non-essential operations so that you can use that excess energy to either fight a threat off or run away from it, something that's decidedly unhelpful if you're stressing about a minor matter that you can neither avoid nor fight against (Madison & Kiecolt-Glaser, 2019).

While your body produces more cortisol when stressed, it produces less prostaglandin, an enzyme that ordinarily reduces the acidity levels of your stomach. This damages your gut microbiome by killing off various microbiota. It also triggers stress-related muscle spasms, which understandably cause you some pain. Furthermore, stress is something that makes you more sensitive to the sensations you feel, which means it makes such pain even more intense and unpleasant. Should all this go on for extended periods of time, then it's inevitable that you'll develop other conditions like IBD as a result of the inflammation that starts flaring up across your intestines.

Adopting healthy stress management techniques is an excellent way of mitigating your risk of experiencing things like this. A helpful technique for managing stress is the 2:1 Breathing Technique, which originates from a form of yoga practice. This makes sense because yoga is known to be effective in reducing stress levels. 2:1 Breathing is a relatively simple technique. All you have to do is exhale for a period of time that's twice as long as you've spent inhaling. For instance, if you breathe in for four seconds, you should breathe out for eight seconds or so (Clarke, n.d.). Though this might not sound like much, its effects on the body and your stress levels are pretty immediate. It instantly starts slowing your heart and breathing rates down, making your sympathetic nervous system less active. Instead, it activates your parasympathetic nervous system, which is the nervous system that's supposed to light up when you're relaxing. One of the things it's in charge of is telling your heart to stop beating so fast, for example.

To practice 2:1 Breathing, sit down in a comfortable seat or lie down and try not to fall asleep in the process. Then slowly inhale and count as you go. Once you're done, slowly exhale, counting yet again, except this time, make sure your exhale time is double that of your inhale time. After you establish a steady rhythm, change up your inhalation-exhalation times for every three breaths. If you inhaled for three seconds and exhaled for six during your first three breaths, go for four seconds and eight seconds in your next three breaths. Afterward, go back to a three-count breath and keep switching things up like that. Keep going until you feel relaxed and are certain that your stress has completely ebbed away.

Another technique to help you relax is performing stretches that can help reduce your stress levels. Stretches like this can be a great way to start and end the day, though you can use them whenever you feel your stress levels spiking up. Stretches are effective for stress relief because they help you release the tension in your muscles. Another benefit of physical activities is that they allow us to release the extra energy stored in our bodies, which we often cannot release due to our predominantly desk-bound, sedentary lifestyles (Migala, 2020). There are three stretches that you can try that can be particularly helpful to you. These are the child's pose, seated spinal twist, and chest opener stretch.

The child's pose is one of the easiest stretches to perform. To start, you'll have to kneel with your feet together and your butt planted on your heels. Spread your knees a little—forming a kind of "V"— and then slowly walk your hands in front of you until your chest is low to the ground. This will be very good for releasing tension from your lower back and actually help improve the quality of your sleep, at least according to the most recent studies (Wei, 2015).

The seated spinal twist is great for when you have to spend long hours in a seated position for work. It releases tension from your spine and helps with your posture. Start by sitting on the edge of your seat with your feet planted firmly on the ground, and then put your right hand on the back of your seat. Place your left hand on your right thigh, then inhale to lengthen your spine. As you exhale, slowly twist your torso back so that you can look over your right shoulder. Hold the pose for a little bit, feel the stretch, and then repeat with your other side (Migala, 2020).

The chest opener is another good stretch for your posture and releases tension from your chest. In the process, it improves oxygen circulation throughout your body. To start, get to your feet and stand with them shoulder-length apart. Clasp your hands behind your back, then push your upper shoulder blades together. This move will push out your chest and expand your lungs.

Your Activity Level Matters

Exercise (as in your level of daily activity) affects your gut microbiome in some fascinating ways. Scientists have found that regular exercise affects the amount of healthy bacteria that reside in your gut. In other words, exercise makes for a more diverse microbiome. It especially increases the sizes of the Oscillospira, Faecalibacterium prausnitzii, Coprococcus, and Lachnospira colonies in your microbiome. It also impacts the number of Firmicutes found there. Clear evidence of this is professional athletes, who tend to have the most diverse microbiomes in today's population (Clauss et al., 2021).

That's not all, though. Aside from increasing your microbiome biodiversity, leading an active lifestyle increases your gut microbiota's respiration levels, which promotes gut health and healthy body functions. This is because higher respiration levels mean producing greater quantities of butyrate, short-chain fatty acids, and other useful enzymes and chemicals. Among these chemicals, butyrate is especially important since it's the fuel source that the cells making up your gut lining need in order to do their job well. When your butyrate levels go down, your gut becomes leakier because those cells become malnourished.

Intestinal Exercises For Your Gut

Speaking of exercise, did you know that there are specific ones you can do for your gut health? These are primarily lower-body exercises that assist your digestion by working your abdominal muscles and getting your digestive system moving. Such exercises can be great for dealing with things like abdominal pain (particularly when they're related to any digestive issues), though they've been known to also help with things like menstrual cramps.

The first exercise that pops to mind when you talk about working your abdominal muscles is sit-ups, which is one of the best intestinal exercises you can do (*5 Exercises That Aid in Optimal Digestive Health*, 2022). This is because they strengthen both your lower and upper abdominal muscles, making them better able to support your digestive system as it works. Abdominal exercises like crunches—which are great for working your lower abdominal muscles particularly—and sit-ups must only be done on an empty stomach. This way, you'll be able to prevent them from damaging your guts in any way.

The second exercise you should do for your digestive health is taking regular walks, as surprising as that might sound. Walking is one of the easiest things you can ever do and one of the best possible exercises out there. This is because it gets all the muscles and systems surrounding your digestive system active and working. In the process, it strengthens your GI tract's ability to contract and relax, which is necessary for the work it needs to do. As a result, it reduces any cramping or bloating you might experience and does away with potential gassiness.

Conclusion

As you've seen throughout the Gut-Brain Connection, your gut microbiome is truly a wondrous thing. A vast and complex system that has been a part of you before you were even born, your gut microbiome plays a crucial role in your health and general well-being. Your gut microbiome can do wonders, from boosting your immune system to aiding in food digestion, improving your mood, and enhancing your memory.

This only holds true, though, if you take care of your gut microbiome in the same way that it takes care of you and how it deserves to be taken care of. As you've seen, this entails doing some very specific things, like maintaining a certain kind of diet so that you can provide your gut microbiota with the micronutrients they need. It further means taking prebiotics and probiotics to strengthen your microbiome and increase its diversity while avoiding eating food that could hurt the helpful microbiota in your gut. It even means leading a more active style if possible. You might not think stretching for just a couple of minutes per day, getting the sleep you need, and taking a 10-minute-long walk every day would make that much of a difference for your gut microbiome. However, you would be wrong, as you've no doubt already come to realize.

The simple fact of the matter is that your second brain, meaning your gut, may very well hold the key to living a long, healthy, and happy life. Again, that's contingent on your ability and willingness to take care of it. The question you need to ask yourself isn't whether it's important to keep your gut healthy. It's what kind of life you want to lead and whether or not you're ready to take the first steps necessary to ensure that you're able to live it well.

References

Adam-Perrot, A., Gutton, L., Sanders, L., & Bouvier, S. (2009). Resistant Starch and Starch-Derived Oligosaccharides as Prebiotics. *Prebiotics and Probiotics Science and Technology*, 259–291. https://doi.org/10.1007/978-0-387-79058-9_9

Adult obesity facts. (2021, February 11). Centers for Disease Control and Prevention. https://www.cdc.gov/obesity/data/adult.html

Akbari, E., Asemi, Z., Daneshvar Kakhaki, R., Kouchaki, E., Bahman, F., Reza Tamtaji, O., Hamidi, G. A., & Salami, M. (2201). Effect of Probiotic Supplementation on Cognitive Function and Metabolic Status in Alzheimer's Disease: A Randomized, Double-Blind and Controlled Trial. *Frontiers Aging Neuroscience*, 8. https://www.frontiersin.org/articles/10.3389/fnag i.2016.00256/full

Akbarian, M., Khani, A., Eghbalpour, S., & Uversky, V. N. (2022). Bioactive Peptides: Synthesis, Sources, Applications, and Proposed Mechanisms of Action. *International Journal of Molecular Sciences*,

23(3), 1445. https://doi.org/10.3390/ijms23031445

Al Bander, Z., Nitert, M. D., Mousa, A., & Naderpoor, N. (2020). The Gut Microbiota and Inflammation: An Overview. *International Journal of Environmental Research and Public Health*, 17(20). https://doi.org/10.3390/ijerph17207618

Alpha-linolenicacid (ALA): Overview, uses, side effects, precautions, interactions, dosing and reviews. (n.d.). WebMD. https://www.webmd.com/vitamins/ai/ingredient mono-1035/alpha-linolenic-acid-ala#:~:text=Alpha%2Dlinolenic%20acid%20(ALA)%20is%20an%20essential%20omega%2D

Alsegiani, A. S., & Shah, Z. A. (2022). The influence of gut microbiota alteration on age-related neuroinflammation and cognitive decline. *Neural Regeneration Research*, 17(11), 2407–2412. https://doi.org/10.4103/1673-5374.335837

Anhê, F. F., Pilon, G., Roy, D., Desjardins, Y., Levy, E., & Marette, A. (2016). TriggeringAkkermansiawith dietary polyphenols: A new weapon to combat the metabolic syndrome? *Gut Microbes*, 7(2), 146–153. https://doi.org/10.1080/19490976.2016.1142036

Anthony, K. (2018, August 16). *SIBO diet 101: What you should and shouldn't eat.* Healthline Media. https://www.healthline.com/health/sibo-diet

Appleton, J. (2018). The Gut-Brain Axis: Influence of Microbiota on Mood and Mental Health. *Integrative Medicine: A Clinician's Journal*, 17(4), 28–32. https://www.ncbi.nlm.nih.gov/pmc/articles/PMC 6469458/

Arentsen, T., Raith, H., Qian, Y., Forssberg, H., & Heijtz, R. D. (2015). Host microbiota modulates development of social preference in mice. *Microbial Ecology in Health & Disease*, 26(0). https://doi.org/10.3402/mehd.v26.29719

Bathina, S., & Das, U. N. (2015). Brain-derived neurotrophic factor and its clinical implications. *Archives of Medical Science*, 11(6), 1164–1178. https://doi.org/10.5114/aoms.2015.56342

Bayliss, J. A., & Andrews, Z. B. (2013). Ghrelin is neuroprotective in Parkinson's disease: molecular mechanisms of metabolic neuroprotection. *Therapeutic Advances in Endocrinology and Metabolism*, 4(1), 25–36. https://doi.org/10.1177/2042018813479645

Bian, X., Chi, L., Gao, B., Tu, P., Ru, H., & Lu, K. (2017). The artificial sweetener acesulfame potassium affects the gut microbiome and body weight gain in CD-1 mice. *PLOS ONE*, 12(6), e0178426. https://doi.org/10.1371/journal.pone.0178426

Bifidobacerium animalis subsp. lactis: Overview, uses, side effects, precautions, interactions, dosing and reviews. (n.d.). WebMD. https://www.webmd.com/vitamins/ai/ingredient mono-891/bifidobacterium-animalis-subsp-lactis#:~:text=People%20use%20B.

Bifidobacterium breve: Overview, uses, side effects, precautions, interactions, dosing and reviews. (n.d.). WebMD. https://www.webmd.com/vitamins/ai/ingredient mono-1665/bifidobacterium-breve#:~:text=breve)%20is%20a%20type%20of

Bishehsari, F., Voigt, R. M., & Keshavarzian, A. (2020). Circadian rhythms and the gut microbiota: from metabolic syndrome to cancer. *Nature Reviews Endocrinology,* 16(12), 731–739. https://doi.org/10.1038/s41574-020-00427-4

Body mass index (BMI). (2020, May 19). Centers for Disease Control and Prevention. https://www.cdc.gov/healthyweight/assessing/b mi/index.html#:~:text=Body%20Mass%20Index %20(BMI)%20is

Boehme, M., Guzzetta, K. E., Wasén, C., & Cox, L. M. (2022). The gut microbiota is an emerging target for improving brain health during aging. *Gut Microbiome,* 1–43. https://doi.org/10.1017/gmb.2022.11

Bourrie, B. C. T., Willing, B. P., & Cotter, P. D. (2016). The Microbiota and Health Promoting Characteristics of the Fermented Beverage Kefir. *Frontiers in Microbiology,* 7. https://doi.org/10.3389/fmicb.2016.00647

Boyers, L. (2022, May 27). *If your gut health is out of whack, you could be missing these important foods.* Mind Body Green. https://www.mindbodygreen.com/articles/gut-health-diet

Breit, S., Kupferberg, A., Rogler, G., & Hasler, G. (2018). Vagus Nerve as Modulator of the Brain–Gut Axis in Psychiatric and Inflammatory Disorders. *Frontiers in Psychiatry,* 9(44). https://doi.org/10.3389/fpsyt.2018.00044

Brown, E. M., Clardy, J., & Xavier, R. J. (2023). Gut microbiome lipid metabolism and its impact on host physiology. *Cell Host & Microbe,* 31(2), 173–186. https://doi.org/10.1016/j.chom.2023.01.009

Brown, V., Sexton, J. A., & Johnston, M. (2006). A Glucose Sensor in Candida albicans. *Eukaryotic Cell,* 5(10), 1726–1737. https://doi.org/10.1128/ec.00186-06

Bryant, E. (2019, October 11). *Gut microbes affect harmful compounds in red meat.* National Institutes of Health (NIH). https://www.nih.gov/news-events/nih-research-matters/gut-microbes-affect-harmful-

compound-red-
meat#:~:text=Research%20has%20shown%20that
%20changes

Burkhart, A. (2020, December 24). *The sucrose intolerance diet: How to get started.* Amy Burkhart. https://theceliacmd.com/the-sucrose-intolerance-diet/

Cadman, B. (2018, October 1). *The 19 best prebiotic foods suitable for vegans.* Medical News Today. https://www.medicalnewstoday.com/articles/323 214#takeaway

Cammann, D., Lu, Y., Cummings, M. J., Zhang, M. L., Cue, J. M., Do, J., Ebersole, J., Chen, X., Oh, E. C., Cummings, J. L., & Chen, J. (2023). Genetic correlations between Alzheimer's disease and gut microbiome genera. *Scientific Reports*, 13(1). https://doi.org/10.1038/s41598-023-31730-5

Carpenter, S. (2012, September). *That gut feeling.* American Psychological Association. https://www.apa.org/monitor/2012/09/gut-feeling

Cheng, W. Y., Wu, C.-Y., & Yu, J. (2020). The role of gut microbiota in cancer treatment: friend or foe? *Gut*, 69(10), 1867–1876. https://doi.org/10.1136/gutjnl-2020-321153

Chong, L. (2019, March 22). *Who should avoid fructans?* Health.osu.edu. https://health.osu.edu/wellness/exercise-and-nutrition/should-you-be-avoiding-fructans#:~:text=Fructans%20can%20be%20a%20Obeneficial

Clapp, M., Aurora, N., Herrera, L., Bhatia, M., Wilen, E., & Wakefield, S. (2017). Gut microbiota's effect on mental health: the gut-brain axis. *Clinics and Practice*, 7(4). https://doi.org/10.4081/cp.2017.987

Clarke, J. (n.d.). *Soothe your nervous system with 2-to-1 breathing.* Yoga International. https://yogainternational.com/article/view/soothe-your-nervous-system-with-2-to-1-breathing/

Clauss, M., Gérard, P., Mosca, A., & Leclerc, M. (2021). Interplay Between Exercise and Gut Microbiome in the Context of Human Health and Performance. *Frontiers Nutrition*, 8. https://www.frontiersin.org/articles/10.3389/fnut.2021.637010/full

Costantini, L., Molinari, R., Farinon, B., & Merendino, N. (2017). Impact of Omega-3 Fatty Acids on the Gut Microbiota. *International Journal of Molecular Sciences*, 18(12), 2645. https://doi.org/10.3390/ijms18122645

Cresci, G. (2022, March 14). What are prebiotics and what do they do? Cleveland Clinic.

https://health.clevelandclinic.org/what-are-prebiotics/

Cronin, P., Joyce, S. A., O'Toole, P. W., & O'Connor, E. M. (2021). Dietary Fibre Modulates the Gut Microbiota. *Nutrients*, 13(5), 1655. https://doi.org/10.3390/nu13051655

Davis, C. D. (2016). The Gut Microbiome and Its Role in Obesity. *Nutrition Today*, 51(4), 167–174. https://doi.org/10.1097/nt.0000000000000167

Depressive disorder (depression). (2023, March 31). World Health Organization. https://www.who.int/news-room/fact-sheets/detail/depression#:~:text=An%20estimated%203.8%25%20of%20the

Diabetes. (2023). World Health Organisation; WHO. https://www.who.int/news-room/fact-sheets/detail/diabetes

Diet, lifestyle and medicines- Irritable bowel syndrome (IBD). (2019). National Health Services. https://www.nhs.uk/conditions/irritable-bowel-syndrome-IBD/diet-lifestyle-and-medicines/

Dietary supplements - Probiotics. (2017). National Institutes of Health. https://ods.od.nih.gov/factsheets/Probiotics-HealthProfessional/

DiMeglio, D., & Mattes, R. (2000). Liquid versus solid carbohydrate: effects on food intake and body weight. *International Journal of Obesity*, 24(6), 794–800. https://doi.org/10.1038/sj.ijo.0801229

Dinan, T. G., & Cryan, J. F. (2012). Regulation of the stress response by the gut microbiota: Implications for psychoneuroendocrinology. *Psychoneuroendocrinology*, 37(9), 1369–1378. https://doi.org/10.1016/j.psyneuen.2012.03.007

Dinan, T. G., Stanton, C., & Cryan, J. F. (2013). Psychobiotics: A Novel Class of Psychotropic. *Biological Psychiatry*, 74(10), 720–726. https://doi.org/10.1016/j.biopsych.2013.05.001

Edermaniger, L. (2021, June 17). Firmicutes bacteria: What are they and why are they important? Atlas Biomed Blog. https://atlasbiomed.com/blog/guide-to-firmicutes/

Eicosapentaenoic acid (EPA) information. (n.d.). Mount Sinai Health System. https://www.mountsinai.org/health-library/supplement/eicosapentaenoic-acid-epa#:~:text=Omega%2D3%20fatty%20acids%20are

Eliza, W. L. Y., Fai, C. K., & Chung, L. P. (2012). Efficacy of Yun Zhi (Coriolus versicolor) on survival in cancer patients: systematic review and

meta-analysis. *Recent Patents on Inflammation &*
Allergy Drug Discovery, 6(1), 78–87.
https://doi.org/10.2174/187221312798889310

Farah, T. (2022, March 4). *The microbiome impacts sleep*
quality, and vice versa. Discover Magazine.
https://www.discovermagazine.com/health/the-
microbiome-impacts-sleep-quality-and-vice-versa

Fazzaura Putri, S. S., Koibuchi, N., Irfannuddin, I.,
Murti, K., Darmawan, H., & Yudianita . (2023,
May 16). The role of gut microbiota on cognitive
development in rodents: a meta-analysis. *The*
Journal of Physiological Sciences Volume.
https://link.springer.com/article/10.1186/s12576-
023-00869-1

Fecal transplant. (2022, April 4). John's Hopkins
Medicine.
https://www.hopkinsmedicine.org/health/treatme
nt-tests-and-therapies/fecal-
transplant#:~:text=Fecal%20transplantation%20is
%20a%20procedure

Ferranti, E. P., Dunbar, S. B., Dunlop, A. L., & Corwin,
E. J. (2014). 20 Things You Didn't Know About
the Human Gut Microbiome. *The Journal of*
Cardiovascular Nursing, 29(6), 479–481.
https://doi.org/10.1097/jcn.0000000000000166

Fessl, S. (2022, May 5). *What happens to the gut microbiome*
after taking antibiotics? The Scientist Magazine®.

https://www.the-scientist.com/news-opinion/what-happens-to-the-gut-microbiome-after-taking-antibiotics-69970#:~:text=He%20describes%20the%20gut%20microbiome

5 exercises that aid in optimal digestive health. (2022, May 18). Allied Digestive Health. https://allieddigestivehealth.com/5-exercises-that-aid-in-optimal-digestive-health/

Francqueville, A. G. de. (2022, March 28). *Gut microbiota may explain some yogurt benefits.* Yogurt in Nutrition. https://www.yogurtinnutrition.com/could-some-benefits-of-yogurt-be-linked-to-gut-microbiota/#:~:text=They%20found%20that%20eating%20yogurt

Galacto-oligosacchardies (GOS): Overview, uses, side effects, precautions, interactions, dosing and reviews. (n.d.). WebMD. https://www.webmd.com/vitamins/ai/ingredient mono-1462/galacto-oligosaccharides-gos#:~:text=Giving%20a%20formula%20that%20contains

Gao, H., Li, X., Chen, X., Hai, D., Wei, C., Zhang, L., & Li, P. (2022). The Functional Roles of Lactobacillus acidophilus in Different Physiological and Pathological Processes. *Journal of Microbiology and Biotechnology*, 32(10), 1226–1233. https://doi.org/10.4014/jmb.2205.05041

Green, E. (2019). Genome. Genome.gov. https://www.genome.gov/genetics-glossary/Genome

Grice, E. A., & Segre, J. A. (2012). The Human Microbiome: Our Second Genome. *Annual Review of Genomics and Human Genetics*, 13(1), 151–170. https://doi.org/10.1146/annurev-genom-090711-163814

Gut Healing Chicken Soup. (2020a, February 25). Katie Stewart - Acne Nutritionist. https://katiestewartwellness.com/2020/02/25/gut-healing-chicken-soup/

Gut healing chicken soup. (2020b, February 25). Katie Stewart | Acne Nutritionist. https://katiestewartwellness.com/2020/02/25/gut-healing-chicken-soup/

Gut health. (n.d.). What about Wheat? Retrieved May 24, 2023, from https://whataboutwheat.ca/nutrition-research-old/gut-health/#:~:text=Eating%20whole%20grains%2C%20like%20wheat

Han, H., Wang, M., Zhong, R., Yi, B., Schroyen, M., & Zhang, H.-F. (2022). Depletion of Gut Microbiota Inhibits Hepatic Lipid Accumulation in High-Fat

Diet-Fed Mice. *International Journal of Molecular Sciences,* 23(16), 9350–9350. https://doi.org/10.3390/ijms23169350

Harmon, K. (2012, June 13). *Saturated fats change gut bacteria and may raise risk for inflammatory bowel disease.* Scientific American Blog Network. https://blogs.scientificamerican.com/observations /saturated-fats-change-gut-bacteria-and-may-raise-risk-for-inflammatory-bowel-disease/

Hathaway, B. (2018, December 17). *Sugar targets gut microbes linked to lean and healthy people.* YaleNews. https://news.yale.edu/2018/12/17/sugar-targets-gut-microbe-linked-lean-and-healthy-people

Hecht, M. (2022, January 27). *6 most common types of probiotics.* Healthline. https://www.healthline.com/health/types-of-probiotics#common-probiotics

Higuera, V. (2022, April 25). Brain fog: 6 potential causes. Healthline. https://www.healthline.com/health/brain-fog#what-is-brain-fog

Huang, T.-T., Lai, J.-B., Du, Y.-L., Xu, Y., Ruan, L.-M., & Hu, S.-H. (2019). Current Understanding of Gut Microbiota in Mood Disorders: An Update of Human Studies. *Frontiers in Genetics,* 10. https://doi.org/10.3389/fgene.2019.00098

Jana, U. K., Kango, N., & Pletschke, B. (2021). Hemicellulose-Derived Oligosaccharides: Emerging Prebiotics in Disease Alleviation. *Frontiers in Nutrition*, 8. https://doi.org/10.3389/fnut.2021.670817

Jandhyala, S. M. (2015). Role of the normal gut microbiota. *World Journal of Gastroenterology*, 21(29), 8787. https://doi.org/10.3748/wjg.v21.i29.8787

Jasirwan, C. O. M., Lesmana, C. R. A., Hasan, I., Sulaiman, A. S., & Gani, R. A. (2019). The role of gut microbiota in non-alcoholic fatty liver disease: pathways of mechanisms. *Bioscience of Microbiota, Food and Health*, 38(3), 81–88. https://doi.org/10.12938/bmfh.18-032

Jayachandran, M., Xiao, J., & Xu, B. (2017). A Critical Review on Health Promoting Benefits of Edible Mushrooms through Gut Microbiota. *International Journal of Molecular Sciences,* 18(9), 1934. https://doi.org/10.3390/ijms18091934

Jennifer A. Fulcher, Fan Li, Nicole H. Tobin, Sara Zabih, Elliott, J., Clark, J. L., D'Aquila, R., Mustanski, B., Kipke, M. D., Shoptaw, S., Gorbach, P. M., & Aldrovandi, G. M. (2022). Gut dysbiosis and inflammatory blood markers precede HIV with limited changes after early seroconversion. *EBio Medicine - the Lancet*, 84.

https://www.thelancet.com/journals/ebiom/articl e/PIIS2352-3964(22)00468-6/fulltext

Johnson, J. (2018, August 22). *Hypothalamus: Function, hormones, and disorders.* Medical News Today. https://www.medicalnewstoday.com/articles/312 628

Johnson, N., Johnson, C. R., Thavarajah, P., Kumar, S., & Thavarajah, D. (2020). The roles and potential of lentil prebiotic carbohydrates in human and plant health. *PLANTS, PEOPLE, PLANET,* 2(4), 310–319. https://doi.org/10.1002/ppp3.10103

JoJack, B. (2023, January 12). *Type 2 diabetes: Healthy gut microbiome linked to insulin response.* Medical News Today. https://www.medicalnewstoday.com/articles/type -2-diabetes-gut-bacteria-linked-to-insulin- sensitivity#The-role-of-the-gut-microbiome

Juber, M. (2022, November 29). *Health benefits of DHA.* WebMD. https://www.webmd.com/diet/health- benefits-dhav

Kang, D.-W., Adams, J. B., Coleman, D. M., Pollard, E. L., Maldonado, J., McDonough-Means, S., Caporaso, J. G., & Krajmalnik-Brown, R. (2019). Long-term benefit of Microbiota Transfer Therapy on autism symptoms and gut microbiota. *Scientific Report*s, 9(1). https://doi.org/10.1038/s41598-019- 42183-0

Kasprzak-Drozd, K., Oniszczuk, T., Stasiak, M., & Oniszczuk, A. (2021). Beneficial Effects of Phenolic Compounds on Gut Microbiota and Metabolic Syndrome. *International Journal of Molecular Sciences*, 22(7), 3715. https://doi.org/10.3390/ijms22073715

Kazemian, N., Mahmoudi, M., Halperin, F., Wu, J. C., & Pakpour, S. (2020). Gut microbiota and cardiovascular disease: opportunities and challenges. *Microbiome*, 8(1). https://doi.org/10.1186/s40168-020-00821-0

Kim, G.-H., Lee, K., & Shim, J. O. (2023). Gut Bacterial Dysbiosis in Irritable Bowel Syndrome: a Case-Control Study and a Cross-Cohort Analysis Using Publicly Available Data Sets. *Microbiology Spectrum*, 11(1). https://doi.org/10.1128/spectrum.02125-22

Kodio, A., Menu, E., & Ranque, S. (2020). Eukaryotic and Prokaryotic Microbiota Interactions. *Microorganisms*, 8(12), 2018. https://doi.org/10.3390/microorganisms8122018

Lecuit, M., & Eloit, M. (2017). The Viruses of the Gut Microbiota. The Microbiota in *Gastrointestinal Pathophysiology*, 179–183. https://doi.org/10.1016/b978-0-12-804024-9.00021-5

Leech, J. (2018, September 24). *9 evidence-based health benefits of kefir.* Healthline Media. https://www.healthline.com/nutrition/9-health-benefits-of-kefir#TOC_TITLE_HDR_6

Leeuwendaal, N. K., Cryan, J. F., & Schellekens, H. (2021). Gut peptides and the microbiome: focus on ghrelin. *Current Opinion in Endocrinology, Diabetes & Obesity,* 28(2), 243–252. https://doi.org/10.1097/med.0000000000000616

Lewandowska-Pietruszka, Z., Figlerowicz, M., & Mazur-Melewska, K. (2022). The History of the Intestinal Microbiota and the Gut-Brain Axis. *Pathogens,* 11(12), 1540. https://doi.org/10.3390/pathogens11121540

Li, H., Limenitakis, J. P., Greiff, V., Yilmaz, B., Schären, O., Urbaniak, C., Zünd, M., Lawson, M. A. E., Young, I. D., Rupp, S., Heikenwälder, M., McCoy, K. D., Hapfelmeier, S., Ganal-Vonarburg, S. C., & Macpherson, A. J. (2020). Mucosal or systemic microbiota exposures shape the B cell repertoire. *Nature,* 584(7820), 274–278. https://doi.org/10.1038/s41586-020-2564-6

Li, W.-Z., Stirling, K., Yang, J.-J., & Zhang, L. (2020). Gut microbiota and diabetes: From correlation to causality and mechanism. *World Journal of Diabetes,* 11(7), 293–308. https://doi.org/10.4239/wjd.v11.i7.293

Li, Y., Hao, Y., Fan, F., & Zhang, B. (2018). The Role of Microbiome in Insomnia, Circadian Disturbance and Depression. *Frontiers in Psychiatry*, 9. https://doi.org/10.3389/fpsyt.2018.00669

Lillo-Pérez, S., Guerra-Valle, M., Orellana-Palma, P., & Petzold, G. (2021). Probiotics in fruit and vegetable matrices: Opportunities for nondairy consumers. *LWT Food, Science, and Technology*, 151. https://doi.org/10.1016/j.lwt.2021.112106

Limosilactobacillus reuteri: Overview, uses, side effects, precautions, interactions, dosing and reviews. (n.d.). WebMD. https://www.webmd.com/vitamins/ai/ingredient mono-1684/limosilactobacillus-reuteri#:~:text=People%20use%20L.

Litwinowicz, K., Choroszy, M., & Waszczuk, E. (2019). Changes in the composition of the human intestinal microbiome in alcohol use disorder: a systematic review. *The American Journal of Drug and Alcohol Abuse*, 46(1), 4–12. https://doi.org/10.1080/00952990.2019.1669629

Liu, B.-N., Liu, X.-T., Liang, Z.-H., & Wang, J.-H. (2021). Gut microbiota in obesity Manuscript source: Invited manuscript. *World Journal of Gastroenterology*, 27(25), 3837–3850. https://doi.org/10.3748/wjg.v27.i25.3837

Lukeš, J., Stensvold, C. R., Jirků-Pomajbíková, K., & Wegener Parfrey, L. (2015). Are Human Intestinal Eukaryotes Beneficial or Commensals? *PLOS Pathogens*, 11(8), e1005039. https://doi.org/10.1371/journal.ppat.1005039

Madison, A., & Kiecolt-Glaser, J. K. (2019). Stress, depression, diet, and the gut microbiota: human–bacteria interactions at the core of psychoneuroimmunology and nutrition. Current *Opinion in Behavioral Sciences*, 28(3), 105–110. https://doi.org/10.1016/j.cobeha.2019.01.011

Major depression. (2022, January). National Institute of Mental Health (NIMH). https://www.nimh.nih.gov/health/statistics/major-depression#:~:text=disorders%2C%20or%20medication.-

Marchesi, J. R. (2010). Prokaryotic and eukaryotic diversity of the human gut. Advances in *Applied Microbiology*, 72, 43–62. https://doi.org/10.1016/S0065-2164(10)72002-5

Mathur, K., Agrawal, R. K., Nagpure, S., & Deshpande, D. (2020). Effect of artificial sweeteners on insulin resistance among type-2 diabetes mellitus patients. *Journal of Family Medicine and Primary Care*, 9(1), 69–71. https://doi.org/10.4103/jfmpc.jfmpc_329_19

Menni, C., Zierer, J., Pallister, T., Jackson, M. A., Long, T., Mohney, R. P., Steves, C. J., Spector, T. D., & Valdes, A. M. (2017). Omega-3 fatty acids correlate with gut microbiome diversity and production of N-carbamylglutamate in middle aged and elderly women. *Scientific Reports*, 7(1), 1–11. https://doi.org/10.1038/s41598-017-10382-2

Metabolic disorders. (n.d.). Medlineplus.gov. https://medlineplus.gov/metabolicdisorders.html #:~:text=A%20metabolic%20disorder%20occurs %20when

Microbiome. (2019). National Cancer Institute. https://www.cancer.gov/publications/dictionaries /cancer-terms/def/microbiome

Migala, J. (2020, August 10). *Quick stretches for stress relief you can do right now.* Everyday Health. https://www.everydayhealth.com/fitness/quick-stretches-for-stress-relief/

Mishra, S. K., Kang, J.-H., Kim, D.-K., Oh, S. H., & Kim, M. K. (2012). Orally administered aqueous extract of Inonotus obliquus ameliorates acute inflammation in dextran sulfate sodium (DSS)-induced colitis in mice. *Journal of Ethnopharmacology*, 143(2), 524–532. https://doi.org/10.1016/j.jep.2012.07.008

Molteni, R., Barnard, R. J., Ying, Z., Roberts, C. K., & Gómez-Pinilla, F. (2002). A high-fat, refined sugar diet reduces hippocampal brain-derived neurotrophic factor, neuronal plasticity, and learning. *Neuroscience*, 112(4), 803–814. https://doi.org/10.1016/s0306-4522(02)00123-9

Nagano, M., Shimizu, K., Kondo, R., Hayashi, C., Sato, D., Kitagawa, K., & Ohnuki, K. (2010). Reduction of depression and anxiety by 4 weeks Hericium erinaceus intake. Biomedical Research (Tokyo, Japan), 31(4), 231–237. https://doi.org/10.2220/biomedres.31.231

National Center for Biotechnology Information. (2018). *What is an inflammation?* Institute for Quality and Efficiency in Health Care (IQWiG). https://www.ncbi.nlm.nih.gov/books/NBK27929 8/#:~:text=Very%20generally%20speaking%2C% 20inflammation%20is

Nelson, A. (2022, November 10). *Health benefits of chickpeas.* WebMD. https://www.webmd.com/food-recipes/health-benefits-chickpeas#:~:text=Chickpeas%20are%20high%20 in%20dietary

Nguyen, M., & Palm, N. W. (2022). Gut instincts in neuroimmunity from the eighteenth to twenty-first centuries. *Seminars in Immunopathology*, 44(5), 569–579. https://doi.org/10.1007/s00281-022-00948-2

Nikawa, H., Makihira, S., Fukushima, H., Nishimura, H., Ozaki, Y., Ishida, K., Darmawan, S., Hamada, T., Hara, K., Matsumoto, A., Takemoto, T., & Aimi, R. (2004). Lactobacillus reuteri in bovine milk fermented decreases the oral carriage of mutans streptococci. *International Journal of Food Microbiology,* 95(2), 219–223. https://doi.org/10.1016/j.ijfoodmicro.2004.03.006

Non-alcoholic fatty liver disease (NAFLD). (2017, October 19). National Health Services. https://www.nhs.uk/conditions/non-alcoholic-fatty-liver-disease/#:~:text=Non%2Dalcoholic%20fatty%20liver%20disease%20(NAFLD)%20is%20the%20term

Novakovic, M., Rout, A., Kingsley, T., Kirchoff, R., Singh, A., Verma, V., Kant, R., & Chaudhary, R. (2020). Role of gut microbiota in cardiovascular diseases. *World Journal of Cardiology,* 12(4), 110–122. https://doi.org/10.4330/wjc.v12.i4.110

Novkovic, B. (2019, November 29). *9+ benefits of bifidobacterium animalis (B. lactis).* SelfDecode Supplements. https://supplements.selfdecode.com/blog/b-animalis/#:~:text=IBD-

O'Hagan, C., Li, J. V., Marchesi, J. R., Plummer, S., Garaiova, I., & Good, M. A. (2017). Long-term multi-species Lactobacillus and Bifidobacterium dietary supplement enhances memory and changes regional brain metabolites in middle-aged rats. *Neurobiology of Learning and Memory*, 144, 36–47. https://doi.org/10.1016/j.nlm.2017.05.015

Obesity. (2022). World Health Organization. https://www.who.int/health-topics/obesity#tab=tab_1

Obesity and Overweight. (2021, June 9). World Health Organization. https://www.who.int/news-room/fact-sheets/detail/obesity-and-overweight

Okada, Y., Tsuzuki, Y., Yasutake, Y., Maruta, K., Takajo, T., Furuhashi, H., Higashiyama, M., Yoshikawa, K., Hokari, R., Tomita , K., Miura, S., Watanabe, C., Komoto , S., Kurihara, C., & Nagao , S. (2016). Tu2021 Anti-Inflammatory Effect of Novel Probiotic Yeasts Isolated From Japanese "Miso" on DSS-Induced Colitis. *AGA ABSTRACTS*, 150(4). https://doi.org/10.1016/S0016-5085(16)33413-8

Omega-3 Fatty Acids. (2017). National Institutes of Health. https://ods.od.nih.gov/factsheets/Omega3FattyAcids-Consumer/

Orenstein, D. (2021, December 17). *Gut-brain connection in autism.* Harvard Health.

https://hms.harvard.edu/news/gut-brain-connection-autism

Osadchiy, V., Martin, C. R., & Mayer, E. A. (2019). The Gut–Brain Axis and the Microbiome: Mechanisms and Clinical Implications. *Clinical Gastroenterology and Hepatology,* 17(2), 322–332. https://doi.org/10.1016/j.cgh.2018.10.002

Pacheco, D., & Wright, H. (2020, October 29). *The best temperature for sleep: Advice & tips.* Sleep Foundation. https://www.sleepfoundation.org/bedroom-environment/best-temperature-for-sleep#:~:text=The%20best%20room%20temperature%20for

Palsdottir, H. (2018, August 28). *11 probiotic foods that are super healthy.* Healthline. https://www.healthline.com/nutrition/11-super-healthy-probiotic-foods#TOC_TITLE_HDR_2

Paone, P., & Cani, P. D. (2020). Mucus barrier, mucins and gut microbiota: the expected slimy partners? Gut, 69(12), 2232–2243. https://doi.org/10.1136/gutjnl-2020-322260

Pappa, A. (2019, June 14). *Grain free strawberry banana bread muffins.* Abra's Kitchen. https://abraskitchen.com/strawberry-banana-bread-muffins/

Park, K.-Y., Jeong, J.-K., Lee, Y.-E., & Daily, J. W. (2014). Health benefits of kimchi (Korean fermented vegetables) as a probiotic food. *Journal of Medicinal Food*, 17(1), 6–20. https://doi.org/10.1089/jmf.2013.3083

Parkinson's disease. (2022, April 14). National Institute on Aging. https://www.nia.nih.gov/health/parkinsons-disease#:~:text=Parkinson

Pei, R., Liu, X., & Bolling, B. (2020). Flavonoids and gut health. *Current Opinion in Biotechnology*, 61, 153–159. https://doi.org/10.1016/j.copbio.2019.12.018

Petre, A. (2017, June 17). Why miso is incredibly healthy. Healthline. https://www.healthline.com/nutrition/why-miso-is-healthy#TOC_TITLE_HDR_4

Petre, A. (2020, March 13). *8 surprising benefits of sauerkraut (plus how to make it).* Healthline. https://www.healthline.com/nutrition/benefits-of-sauerkraut#2.-Improves-your-digestion

Pinto-Sanchez, M. I., Hall, G. B., Ghajar, K., Nardelli, A., Bolino, C., Lau, J. T., Martin, F.-P., Cominetti, O., Welsh, C., Rieder, A., Traynor, J., Gregory, C., De Palma, G., Pigrau, M., Ford, A. C., Macri, J., Berger, B., Bergonzelli, G., Surette, M. G., & Collins, S. M. (2017). Probiotic Bifidobacterium longum NCC3001 Reduces Depression Scores and

Alters Brain Activity: A Pilot Study in Patients With Irritable Bowel Syndrome. *Gastroenterology*, 153(2), 448-459.e8. https://doi.org/10.1053/j.gastro.2017.05.003

Polo, A., Arora, K., Ameur, H., Di Cagno, R., De Angelis, M., & Gobbetti, M. (2020). Gluten-free diet and gut microbiome. *Journal of Cereal Science*, 95, 103058. https://doi.org/10.1016/j.jcs.2020.103058

Probiotics: What is it, benefits, side effects, food & types. (2020, March 9). Cleveland Clinic. https://my.clevelandclinic.org/health/articles/145 98-probiotics

Radjabzadeh, D., Bosch, J. A., Uitterlinden, A. G., Zwinderman, A. H., Ikram, M. A., van Meurs, J. B. J., Luik, A. I., Nieuwdorp, M., Lok, A., van Duijn, C. M., Kraaij, R., & Amin, N. (2022). Gut microbiome-wide association study of depressive symptoms. *Nature Communications*, 13(1), 7128. https://doi.org/10.1038/s41467-022-34502-3

Raman, R. (2017, May 17). *14 natural ways to improve your insulin sensitivity*. Healthline. https://www.healthline.com/nutrition/improve-insulin-sensitivity#:~:text=Insulin%20sensitivity%20refers%20to%20how

Rao, M., & Gershon, M. D. (2016). The Bowel and beyond: the Enteric Nervous System in

Neurological Disorders. *Nature Reviews Gastroenterology & Hepatology*, 13(9), 517–528. https://doi.org/10.1038/nrgastro.2016.107

Rapson, J. (2018, August 20). *What are the benefits of fermented foods?* Heart Foundation NZ. https://www.heartfoundation.org.nz/about-us/news/blogs/fermented-foods-the-latest-trend

Raypole, C. (2021, January 27). *Trust your gut: What it actually means.* Healthline. https://www.healthline.com/health/mental-health/trust-your-gut#when-to-trust-them

Razak, M. A., Begum, P. S., Viswanath, B., & Rajagopal, S. (2017). Multifarious Beneficial Effect of Nonessential Amino Acid, Glycine: A Review. *Oxidative Medicine and Cellular Longevity*, 2017, 1–8. https://doi.org/10.1155/2017/1716701

Rege, S. (2019, April 22). *The simplified guide to the gut brain axis - How the gut talks to the brain.* Psych Scene Hub. https://psychscenehub.com/psychinsights/the-simplified-guide-to-the-gut-brain-axis/

Ries, J. (2023, January 20). *IBD and gut bacteria: How they're related.* Healthline. https://www.healthline.com/health-news/IBD-and-gut-bacteria-how-theyre-related#The-bottom-line

Rijo-Ferreira, F., & Takahashi, J. S. (2019). Genomics of circadian rhythms in health and disease. *Genome Medicine*, 11(1). https://doi.org/10.1186/s13073-019-0704-0

Roberfroid, M. B. (1997). Health Benefits of Non-Digestible Oligosaccharides. Advances in Experimental *Medicine and Biology*, 211–219. https://doi.org/10.1007/978-1-4615-5967-2_22

Romano, S., Savva, G. M., Bedarf, J. R., Charles, I. G., Hildebrand, F., & Narbad, A. (2021). Meta-analysis of the Parkinson's disease gut microbiome suggests alterations linked to intestinal inflammation. *Npj Parkinson's Disease*, 7(1), 1–13. https://doi.org/10.1038/s41531-021-00156-z

Rush, T., & Barrell, A. (2021, October 5). *Lactic acid: Role in the body and impact on exercise*. Medical News Today. https://www.medicalnewstoday.com/articles/326521#:~:text=Lactic%20acid%20is%20an%20integral

Sadrekarimi, H., Gardanova, Z. R., Bakhshesh, M., Ebrahimzadeh, F., Yaseri, A. F., Thangavelu, L., Hasanpoor, Z., Zadeh, F. A., & Kahrizi, M. S. (2022). Emerging role of human microbiome in cancer development and response to therapy: special focus on intestinal microflora. *Journal of*

Translational   Medicine,   20(1). https://doi.org/10.1186/s12967-022-03492-7

Salas, J. T., & Chang, T. L. (2014). Microbiome in HIV infection. *Clinics in Laboratory Medicine, 34*(4), 733–745. https://doi.org/10.1016/j.cll.2014.08.005

Sandler, R. H., Finegold, S. M., Bolte, E. R., Buchanan, C. P., Maxwell, A. P., Väisänen, M.-L., Nelson, M. N., & Wexler, H. M. (2000). Short-Term Benefit From Oral Vancomycin Treatment of Regressive-Onset Autism. *Journal of Child Neurology, 15*(7), 429–435. https://doi.org/10.1177/088307380001500701

Sanfins, A. (2020, December 2). *Gut bacteria can help rebuild the immune system.* Medical Newst Today. https://www.medicalnewstoday.com/articles/gut-bacteria-can-help-rebuild-the-immune-system

Sanidad, K. Z., Amir, M., Ananthanarayanan, A., Singaraju, A., Shiland, N. B., Hong, H. S., Kamada, N., Inohara, N., Núñez, G., & Zeng, M. Y. (2022). Maternal gut microbiome–induced IgG regulates neonatal gut microbiome and immunity. *Science Immunology,* 7(72). https://doi.org/10.1126/sciimmunol.abh3816

Saranya, M. (2020). Basic anatomy and neuroendocrine pathway of the Pituitary gland. *Journal of Clinical and Molecular Endocrinology, 5*(4). https://clinical-and-molecular-endocrinology.imedpub.com/basic-anatomy-and-neuroendocrine-pathway-of-the-pituitary-gland.php?aid=33610#:~:text=The%20neuroendocrine%20pathways%20are%20a

Schluter, J., Peled, J. U., Taylor, B. P., Markey, K. A., Smith, M., Taur, Y., Niehus, R., Staffas, A., Dai, A., Fontana, E., Amoretti, L. A., Wright, R. J., Morjaria, S., Fenelus, M., Pessin, M. S., Chao, N. J., Lew, M., Bohannon, L., Bush, A., & Sung, A. D. (2020). The gut microbiota is associated with immune cell dynamics in humans. *Nature*, 588(7837), 303–307. https://doi.org/10.1038/s41586-020-2971-8

Schoeler, M., & Caesar, R. (2019). Dietary lipids, gut microbiota and lipid metabolism. *Reviews in Endocrine and Metabolic Disorders*, 20(4), 461–472. https://doi.org/10.1007/s11154-019-09512-0

Sen, P., Molinero-Perez, A., O'Riordan, K. J., McCafferty, C. P., O'Halloran, K. D., & Cryan, J. F. (2021). Microbiota and sleep: awakening the gut feeling. *Trends in Molecular Medicine*, 27(10), 935–945. https://doi.org/10.1016/j.molmed.2021.07.004

Snyder, C. (2021, January 14). *9 surprising benefits of kimchi.* Healthline. https://www.healthline.com/nutrition/benefits-of-kimchi#2.-Contains-probiotics

Strandwitz, P. (2018). Neurotransmitter modulation by the gut microbiota. *Brain Research*, 1693(Pt B), 128–133. https://doi.org/10.1016/j.brainres.2018.03.015

Sudo, N., Chida, Y., Aiba, Y., Sonoda, J., Oyama, N., Yu, X.-N., Kubo, C., & Koga, Y. (2004). Postnatal microbial colonization programs the hypothalamic-pituitary-adrenal system for stress response in mice. *The Journal of Physiology*, 558(1), 263–275. https://doi.org/10.1113/jphysiol.2004.063388

Suez, J., Korem, T., Zeevi, D., Zilberman-Schapira, G., Thaiss, C. A., Maza, O., Israeli, D., Zmora, N., Gilad, S., Weinberger, A., Kuperman, Y., Harmelin, A., Kolodkin-Gal, I., Shapiro, H., Halpern, Z., Segal, E., & Elinav, E. (2014). Artificial sweeteners induce glucose intolerance by altering the gut microbiota. *Nature*, 514(7521), 181–186. https://doi.org/10.1038/nature13793

Szentirmai, É., Millican, N. S., Massie, A. R., & Kapás, L. (2019). Butyrate, a metabolite of intestinal bacteria, enhances sleep. *Scientific Reports*, 9(1). https://doi.org/10.1038/s41598-019-43502-1

Tanaka, M., & Nakayama, J. (2017). Development of the gut microbiota in infancy and its impact on health in later life. *Allergology International*, 66(4), 515–522. https://doi.org/10.1016/j.alit.2017.07.010

Taniya, M. A., Chung, H.-J., Al Mamun, A., Alam, S., Aziz, Md. A., Uddin Emon, N., Islam, Md. M., Hong, 7Seong-Tshool, Podder, B. R., Ara Mimi, A., Aktar Suchi, S., & Xiao, J. (2022). Role of Gut Microbiome in Autism Spectrum Disorder and Its Therapeutic Regulation. *Frontiers in Cellular and Infection Microbiology*, 12. https://www.frontiersin.org/articles/10.3389/fcimb.2022.915701/full

The microbiome. (2017, August 16). The Nutrition Source. https://www.hsph.harvard.edu/nutritionsource/microbiome/#:~:text=In%20addition%20to%20family%20genes

The stages of HIV infection. (2021, August 20). National Institute of Health. https://hivinfo.nih.gov/understanding-hiv/fact-sheets/stages-hiv-infection#:~:text=The%20second%20stage%20of%20HIV

Tresca, A. J. (2021, November 9). *Why do beans cause gas?* Verywell Health. https://www.verywellhealth.com/why-do-beans-cause-gas-1942947#:~:text=Beans%20(legumes)%20cause%20gas%20because

Try a FODMAPs diet to manage irritable bowel syndrome. (2014, October 10). Harvard Health.

https://www.health.harvard.edu/diseases-and-conditions/a-new-diet-to-manage-irritable-bowel-syndrome

Trzeciak, P., & Herbet, M. (2021). Role of the Intestinal Microbiome, Intestinal Barrier and Psychobiotics in Depression. *Nutrients*, 13(3), 927. https://doi.org/10.3390/nu13030927

Type 2 diabetes. (2021, December 16). Centers for Disease Control and Prevention. https://www.cdc.gov/diabetes/basics/type2.html #:~:text=More%20than%2037%20million%20Americans

Uchiyama, J., Akiyama, M., Hase, K., Kumagai, Y., & Kim, Y.-G. (2022). Gut microbiota reinforce host antioxidant capacity via the generation of reactive sulfur species. *Cell Reports*, 38(10), 110479. https://doi.org/10.1016/j.celrep.2022.110479

University of Bern. (2020, August 5). Gut microbes shape our antibodies before we are infected by pathogens. ScienceDaily. https://www.sciencedaily.com/releases/2020/08/200805124038.htm

Varesi, A., Pierella, E., Romeo, M., Piccini, G. B., Alfano, C., Bjørklund, G., Oppong, A., Ricevuti, G., Esposito, C., Chirumbolo, S., & Pascale, A. (2022). The Potential Role of Gut Microbiota in Alzheimer's Disease: From Diagnosis to

Treatment. *Nutrients*, 14(3), 668. https://doi.org/10.3390/nu14030668

Vespa, J. (2021, May 15). *10 minute chickpea tuna salad {easy + healthy}*. Dishing out Health. https://dishingouthealth.com/chickpea-tuna-salad/#recipe

Villines, Z. (2017, July 29). *Free radicals: How do they affect the body?* Medical News Today. https://www.medicalnewstoday.com/articles/318652#How-do-free-radicals-damage-the-body

Vourakis, M., Mayer, G., & Rousseau, G. (2021). The Role of Gut Microbiota on Cholesterol Metabolism in Atherosclerosis. *International Journal of Molecular Sciences*, 22(15), 8074. https://doi.org/10.3390/ijms22158074

Walder, C. (2021, September 20). *Salmon with sweet potato mash & miso coconut sauce*. Walder Wellness. https://www.walderwellness.com/salmon-sweet-potato-mash-miso-coconut-sauce/

Wang, X., Qi, Y., & Zheng, H. (2022). Dietary Polyphenol, Gut Microbiota, and Health Benefits. *Antioxidants*, 11(6), 1212. https://doi.org/10.3390/antiox11061212

Wang, X., Zhang, P., & Zhang, X. (2021). Probiotics Regulate Gut Microbiota: An Effective Method to

Improve Immunity. *Molecules*, 26(19), 6076. https://doi.org/10.3390/molecules26196076

Watson, K. (2019, October 23). *Everything you need to know about flavonoids.* Healthline. https://www.healthline.com/health/what-are-flavonoids-everything-you-need-to-know

Waxenbaum, J. A., Reddy, V., & Varacallo, M. (2020, August 10). Anatomy, Autonomic Nervous System. *PubMed; StatPearls Publishing.* https://www.ncbi.nlm.nih.gov/books/NBK53984 5/#:~:text=The%20autonomic%20nervous%20sy stem%20is

Wei, M. (2015, December 4). *Yoga for better sleep.* Harvard Health Blog. https://www.health.harvard.edu/blog/8753-201512048753

Wernroth, M.-L., Peura, S., Hedman, A. M., Hetty, S., Vicenzi, S., Kennedy, B., Fall, K., Svennblad, B., Andolf, E., Pershagen, G., Theorell-Haglöw, J., Nguyen, D., Sayols-Baixeras, S., Dekkers, K. F., Bertilsson, S., Almqvist, C., Dicksved, J., & Fall, T. (2022). Development of gut microbiota during the first 2 years of life. *Scientific Reports*, 12(1), 9080. https://doi.org/10.1038/s41598-022-13009-3

What is Alzheimer's disease? (2020, June 2). Centers for Disease Control and Prevention.

https://www.cdc.gov/aging/aginginfo/alzheimers.
htm#:~:text=Alzheimer

What is diabetes? (2016, December). National Institute of
Diabetes and Digestive and Kidney Diseases.
https://www.niddk.nih.gov/health-
information/diabetes/overview/what-is-
diabetes#:~:text=Diabetes%20is%20a%20disease
%20that

What is inflammatory bowel disease (IBD)? (2018,
November 9). Centers for Disease Control and
Prevention. https://www.cdc.gov/ibd/what-is-
IBD.htm#:~:text=Inflammatory%20bowel%20dis
ease%20(IBD)%20is

Wongkaew, M., Tangjaidee, P., Leksawasdi, N.,
Jantanasakulwong, K., Rachtanapun, P.,
Seesuriyachan, P., Phimolsiripol, Y., Chaiyaso, T.,
Ruksiriwanich, W., Jantrawut, P., & Sommano, S.
R. (2022). Mango Pectic Oligosaccharides: A Novel
Prebiotic for Functional Food. *Frontiers in Nutrition*,
9. https://doi.org/10.3389/fnut.2022.798543

Xu, H., Luo, J., Huang, J., & Wen, Q. (2018).
Flavonoids intake and risk of type 2 diabetes
mellitus. *Medicine*, 97(19), e0686.
https://doi.org/10.1097/md.0000000000010686

Yang, Y., & Palm, N. W. (2020). Immunoglobulin A
and the microbiome. *Current Opinion in Microbiology*,

56,   89–96.
https://doi.org/10.1016/j.mib.2020.08.003

Zhu, S., Huang, M., Feng, G., Miao, Y., Wo, H., Zeng, M., & Lo, M. (2018). Gelatin versus its two major degradation products, prolyl-hydroxyproline and glycine, as supportive therapy in experimental colitis in mice. *Food, Science, & Nutrition.* https://www.ncbi.nlm.nih.gov/pmc/articles/PMC 6021736/

Made in United States
Troutdale, OR
01/02/2025

27540408R00110